Breast Cancer 4
Advances in Research and Treatment

Breast Cancer
Advances in Research and Treatment

Edited by **WILLIAM L. McGUIRE, M.D.**

A Continuation Order Plan is available for this series. A continuation order will bring delivery of each new volume immediately upon publication. Volumes are billed only upon actual shipment. For further information please contact the publisher.

Breast Cancer 4
Advances in Research and Treatment

Edited by
William L. McGuire, M. D.
University of Texas Health Science Center
San Antonio, Texas

Springer Science+Business Media, LLC

The Library of Congress cataloged the first volume of this title as follows:

Breast cancer. v. 1 –
New York, London, Plenum Medical Book Co., c1977-

v. ill. 24 cm.
Editor: v. 1 –   : W.L. McGuire.

1. Breast–Cancer–Periodicals. I. McGuire, William L.
RC280.B8B66   616.9′94′49   79-646815
                                                              MARC-S

ISBN 978-1-4615-6573-4   ISBN 978-1-4615-6571-0 (eBook)
DOI 10.1007/978-1-4615-6571-0

© 1981 Springer Science+Business Media New York
Originally published by Plenum Press, New York in 1981
Softcover reprint of the hardcover 1st edition 1981
233 Spring Street, New York, N.Y. 10013

Plenum Medical Book Company is an imprint of Plenum Publishing Corporation

Contributors

Benjamin Franklin Byrd, Jr., Nashville, Tennessee 37203

William H. Hartmann, Department of Pathology, Vanderbilt University Hospital, Nashville, Tennessee 37232

W. A. Knight III, Division of Oncology, Department of Medicine, University of Texas Health Science Center, San Antonio, Texas 78284

Rose Kushner, Breast Cancer Advisory Center, Kensington, Maryland 20795

Frederique Kuttenn, Department of Reproductive Endocrinology, Hôpital Necker, 75730 Paris Cedex 15, France

Robert B. Livingston, Department of Hematology and Medical Oncology, Cleveland Clinic, Cleveland, Ohio 44106

Pierre Mauvais-Jarvis, Department of Reproductive Endocrinology, Hôpital Necker, 75730 Paris Cedex 15, France

W. L. McGuire, Division of Oncology, Department of Medicine, University of Texas Health Science Center, San Antonio, Texas 78284

C. K. Osborne, Division of Oncology, Department of Medicine, University of Texas Health Science Center, San Antonio, Texas 78284

Goi Sakamoto, Department of Pathology, Cancer Institute, Tokyo 170, Japan

Regine Sitruk-Ware, Department of Reproductive Endocrinology, Hôpital Necker, 75730 Paris Cedex 15, France

Reuven K. Snyderman, College of Medicine/Dentistry of New Jersey–Rutgers Medical School, University Heights, Piscataway, New Jersey 08854

Haruo Sugano, Cancer Institute, Tokyo 170, Japan

M. G. Yochmowitz, Division of Oncology, Department of Medicine, University of Texas Health Science Center, San Antonio, Texas 78284

Preface

This is the fourth book in a series dealing with breast cancer. Volumes 1-3 were concerned with treatment, experimental biology, and a number of varied timely topics. The present volume continues to review the breast cancer field in the broadest sense.

The first chapter addresses the question of selecting appropriate chemotherapy for the patient. In the 1970s, great advances were seen in our ability to achieve objective tumor regression with empirical combinations of chemotherapeutic agents. The next decade will focus on precise methods to select those agents likely to have the greatest benefit in individual patients. Livingston has provided us with a thorough review of the current state of the art.

We have known for some time that steroid hormone receptor assays of considerable value to clinicians caring for patients with advanced disease. Osborne and colleagues now present considerable arguments that receptor assays are also useful in the setting of primary breast cancer for purposes of both prognosis and treatment strategy.

A very important clinical problem which has received little attention in the research laboratory is benign breast disease. If one inquires about the medical therapy of this disorder in the United States, it is obvious that the majority of physicians would appreciate a better understanding of the pathophysiology which might lead to improved therapies. Mauvais-Jarvis and co-workers provide us with such an account from their wide experience.

The next chapter is a departure from the usual in this series in that a lay person writes about breast cancer from a consumer's point of view. More and more is being written in popular ladies' magazines about breast cancer, but, unfortunately, busy physicians often do not have the time or inclination to read such journals. To present a plausible consumer's point of view to physicians, researchers, and the like, the author must have a very special knowledge of breast cancer or have a very interesting story to tell. Ms. Kushner meets both criteria. Motivated by her own personal experience with breast cancer, she has devoted the majority of her time learning more about the disease and sharing this knowledge with countless numbers of women. Readers of this chapter cannot help but be impressed with her broad understanding of what we know and do not know about breast cancer.

It is some time now since the original implementation of the Breast Cancer Detection Center Projects. From a unique historical perspective, Byrd reviews the thinking and planning that occurred and documents the cooperation between the American Cancer Society and the National Cancer Institute in this effort. The original goals are put into sharp focus and, where possible, the benefits of the program are illustrated.

Much emphasis has been placed on the proper surgical management of primary breast cancer. The role of reconstructive surgery is just now emerging. Snyderman reviews current options as well as an approach to women with a high risk of developing breast cancer.

Epidemiologists have sought clues to the etiology of breast cancer from the well-documented differences in incidence and prognosis between different countries. This is well-illustrated by Sakamoto and colleagues, who detail such differences between patients in Tokyo and Nashville. Although answers to etiology are not provided from this study, the fact that Japanese women with breast cancer have a more favorable prognosis is again demonstrated. Furthermore, the authors suggest that these differences may be disappearing, leading to a more homogeneous worldwide disease.

In summary, Volume 4 of this series covers a broad range of topics, all of which we hope will provide stimulating reading for basic biologists as well as for clinicians caring for patients with breast cancer.

William L. McGuire, M.D.

November, 1980

Contents

5. Breast Cancer Detection Center Projects **151**

Benjamin Franklin Byrd, Jr.

6. Reconstruction of the Female Breast after Mastectomy **185**

Reuven K. Snyderman

Methods to Predict Response to Chemotherapy

ROBERT B. LIVINGSTON

1. General Considerations

There have been numerous attempts to develop an assay system that will allow the correct choice of systemic therapy for an individual patient with cancer. The empirical method used at present to select such therapy involves both the possibility that ineffective agents will be chosen and the probability that the patient will suffer some untoward effects as a result of their use.

1.1. *In Vivo*—Xenograft Systems

The rationale for *in vivo* predictive assays is that human xenografts will retain response characteristics of the original host system. A major requirement for such assays is that the xenograft not be rejected by host-dependent mechanisms, which means that the animal species must be immunosuppressed. This can be accomplished by such techniques as irradiation of the entire animal or by use of an inbred line with inherently defective immune rejection capabilities, such as the nude mouse. The latter is currently more popular.[1] Responsiveness to chemotherapy of xenografts grown in nude mice is now under intensive investigation. At best, however, the nude mouse system has serious limitations: (1) the latent period, before transplanted tumor becomes apparent in the mouse, is 10–31 days or more, and another 3–6 weeks is involved in carrying out *in vivo* assays for chemotherapy effect; (2) metastasis is

---

ROBERT B. LIVINGSTON • Department of Hematology and Medical Oncology, Cleveland Clinic, Cleveland, Ohio 44106.

unusual; (3) growth kinetics of the tumor growing in the nude mouse are different from those in the human host[2]; (4) serial passage alters responsiveness to specific chemotherapy[3]; and (5) to quote Giovanella *et al.* [1]: "Strict sterile techniques must be applied in caring for these animals and meticulous attention given to the preparation of surgical specimens."

1.2. *In Vitro*

Cline[4] has summarized the minimal conditions that must be met for an *in vitro* system to have clinical usefulness. (1) the drug must be active in the form in which it is added to the *in vitro* system or must be converted to an active form by the constituents of the system; (2) the metabolism of the malignant cells *in vivo* and *in vitro* must be sufficiently similar so that drug effects under the two conditions are comparable; (3) there must be sufficient time for drug action to become manifest (but not so long that major changes in the "control" cell population take place, relative to conditions *in vivo*); and (4) a representative sample of tumor must be obtained for testing. To this list should be added a few additional requirements: (5) the drug concentration added must be realistic; (6) the test must be relatively inexpensive, rapid, simple, and reproducible if it is ever to have wide application; and (7) most critically, there must be a strong demonstrated correlation with clinical results. Furthermore, it is more important that such a test be sensitive than that it be specific. Both goals are desirable, but for an *in vitro* test to exclude compounds that are useful *in vivo* is a more serious problem than for it to occasionally overpredict clinical usefulness.

2. *In Vitro* Predictive Systems

A variety of *in vitro* predictive techniques have been employed. They can be considered in five broad categories: (1) those based on primary site of action; (2) those based on primary or secondary changes in cellular metabolism; (3) those based on changes in cell morphology; (4) those based on drug uptake or activation by intact cells; and (5) those based on loss of reproductive integrity.

2.1. Systems Based on Primary Site of Action

2.1.1. *Enzyme Inhibition*

These tests measure the effect of a drug on a defined enzyme or metabolic pathway in isolated tumor cells and correlate this effect with the drug's clinical usefulness. Examples are the ability of L-asparaginase to block asparagine synthesis in sensitive cells,[5] the inhibition of dihydrofolate reductase by methotrexate (MTX),[6] and the effect of 5-fluorouracil (5-FU) on *de novo* thymidine synthesis.[7] Each has been reported to show some correlation with observed clinical outcome. None has, however, been widely adopted or routinely practiced, even by its originators. Tests based on inhibition of an enzymatic pathway usually involve cumbersome and somewhat difficult assay systems. More important as a general criticism is the fact that they are not applicable to drugs the primary site of action of which is unknown or poorly defined as is the case for many chemotherapeutic agents. Finally, they may not be accurate if there are multiple primary sites of drug action, each of varying importance in individual tumors: although MTX and 5-FU have been the major candidates for this type of assay, there is some controversy over the primacy of a single enzyme system in even these cases.[8,9]

2.1.2. Alkylation

Workers in Kohn's laboratory have described a series of experiments in which differences in the formation and removal of DNA cross-links have been examined, both with respect to types of alkylating agent[10] and in terms of sensitive vs. resistant cell lines[11] or xenografts[12] In a sensitive cell line, little or no repair of cross-linking was observed, while the resistant line showed complete repair by 48 hr. In a drug-resistant xenograft tumor, there was substantially less cross-linking at all time points examined than in its sensitive counterpart. These investigations were carried out with a recently developed alkaline elution technique, which has some promise for ultimate clinical application.

2.2. Systems Based on Metabolic Changes

2.2.1. Oxygen Consumption

Tests that measure effects on oxygen consumption have fallen from favor, the reasons being related both to technical difficulties of measurement and to the large amount of variation in this parameter in control cell populations.

2.2.2. Carbohydrate Metabolism

Tests that measure effects on carbohydrate metabolism usually depend on reduction of a dye marker, such as methylene blue; failure to reduce the dye results in a zone of color around "sensitive" cells. Using such an assay system, Di Paolo[13] reported a strong correlation of clinical results with ineffectiveness *in vitro*: 0 of 42 patients responded. Unfortunately, only 12 of 47 patients whose tumors were "sensitive" *in vitro* had clinical effect from the same drugs employed *in vivo*. Kondo,[14] reported similar overall results: a "correct" prediction of effectiveness of chemotherapy for solid tumors in 61–89% of cases, but with the best correlation lying in the prediction of nonresponse. At least in theory, one might expect there to be difficulties with such tests, both because the enzymes of the Krebs cycle are relatively far removed from the probable primary impact of most anticancer drugs and because of the ability of many tumor cells to survive indefinitely under hypoxic conditions.

2.2.3. Membrane Effects

Tests based on the ability to exclude supravital stains have shown minimal effects from *in vitro* exposure to drugs[15]: 5-FU, for example, reduced the "mean viability index" from 87 to 70% on cells from carcinoma of the breast in tissue culture. It is now well established that a cell may be profoundly damaged and incapable of reproduction, yet still be capable of excluding supravital stains.[16-18] Thus, it appears that as an endpoint for drug effect, loss of dye exclusion is too insensitive to provide the desired correlation with loss of reproductive potential.

^{51}Cr has been used extensively in immunological assays for cytotoxicity[19]; it is thought that ^{51}Cr is covalently bound to basic amino acids of intracellular proteins,[20] which leak from the cell as a consequence of membrane damage. The extent of the target-cell damage is therefore assessed as a function of ^{51}Cr release. There is little reported experience with the use of this assay as an indicator of drug effects from chemotherapy; the one available study[21] found that "the degree of release was so modest that this assay appeared completely insensitive in measuring the magnitude of injury caused by chemotherapeutic agents." Like dye exclusion tests, ^{51}Cr release assays are probably dependent on the loss of cell-membrane integrity; although this may be a relatively early event in the interaction of tumor target cells and host killer cells, it probably is not a sensitive indicator of lethal drug damage.

2.2.4. RNA Synthesis

Effects on RNA synthesis have been assessed by several investigators and compared with clinical results. Cline[22] found that depression of [^{3}H]uridine incorporation into leukemic blasts by more than 50%

after *in vitro* exposure for approximately 24 hr to cortisol at concentrations of 5×10^{-5} or 5×10^{-6} M, or more than 90% inhibition with vincristine at 7×10^{-5} M, was highly correlated with *in vivo* cytotoxicity. Depression of [³H]thymidine incorporation appeared to correlate equally well with cortisol, was not studied for vincristine, and showed a better correlation with *in vitro* cytotoxicity than effects on [³H]uridine incorporation for the drug cytosine arabinoside (ARA-C). The drug concentrations that produced *in vitro* effects were much higher than those achievable pharmacologically.

2.2.5. DNA Synthesis

Among those who have measured both effects on uridine incorporation into RNA and effects on thymidine or formate incorporation into DNA, results vary with regard to their relative predictive efficacy. Wayss et al,[23] using a short period of drug exposure to tumor cells *in vitro* (2 hr), and correlating results with observed antitumor effects in several animal systems, concluded that depression of RNA synthesis was more useful, since there were no false-negative predictions based on uridine incorporation into RNA, and false-negative predictions did occur for the efficacy of actinomycin D, based on tracer incorporation into DNA. However, both systems predicted for *in vivo* efficacy of adriamycin in all tumors studied. Kaufman,[24] on the other hand, found that inhibition of thymidine uptake *in vitro* was greater than that of uridine uptake into cell suspensions, using 4-hydroperoxycyclophosphamide in the sensitive Walker 256 carcinosarcoma. Bickiss et al,[25] and Wolberg and Brown[26.27] reported significant correlation of clinical response with depression of DNA synthesis *in vitro*, after 2-hr and 24-hr incubation with tumor cells, respectively using fluorinated pyrimidines as well as other compounds. Knock et al,[28] using the longer 24-hr period of incubation with drugs, also felt that depression of DNA synthesis was the more significant parameter. Zittoun et al,[29] using a 2-hr period of drug incubation with leukemic blasts, had results at variance with those of Cline; no parallel was seen between depression of thymidine incorporation and that of uridine, and they "did not observe any prognostic value in the latter."

Overall, the weight of available evidence seems to favor use of a measure of depression of DNA synthesis over one of RNA synthesis, as an endpoint for *in vitro* effects to correlate with clinical efficacy. At least for proliferating cells, it seems logical that depression of DNA synthesis should be a common manifestation of cell damage leading to loss of reproductive integrity, regardless of the primary mechanism of action. For most chemotherapeutic agents, proliferating cells are preferentially affected; thus, a test that measures effects on DNA synthesis could be reasonably expected to correlate with drug efficacy, provided the other criteria for clinical usefulness are met. The interpretation of [^{3}H]uridine incorporation, on the other hand, is difficult because of the complexity of control of RNA synthesis, the turnover of unstable RNA fractions,[30] and the resultant possibility that changes in RNA synthesis may or may not be associated with loss of reproductive potential.

2.3. Systems Based on Morphological Changes

2.3.1. Semiquantitative

In vitro predictive tests that depend on the interpretation of morphological changes in tumor cells, even when efforts are made to make such interpretations semiquantitative,[31] appear unpromising; there is always a subjective element, interpretation of changes is technically demanding and requires experience, and clinical correlations to date have been disappointing. Hurley and Yount,[32] using semiquantitative criteria for assessing cell damage, found that only 50% of 373 specimens used were satisfactory; among these, 35% showed a negative correlation (usually positive effect in vitro and no benefit in vivo).

2.3.2. Chromosome Condensation

Hittelman and Rao[33] recently described an assay system for prediction of response in acute leukemia, based on a special kind of "morphological change"; it involves measurement of the fraction of prematurely condensed chromosomes apparent in bone marrow cells that have been fused with mitotic Chinese hamster ovary cells by the Sendai virus technique. This fraction, thought to represent those cells with proliferative potential (late G_1, S, and G_2), was decreased by chemotherapy in vivo among patients who were destined to achieve remission and unaffected by such chemotherapy in nonresponders. Whether the technique could be applied to an in vitro exposure type of predictive system, or to a morphologically heterogeneous solid tumor system, remains to be determined.

2.4. Systems Based on Drug Uptake or Activation

The work of Kessel and others[34-37] with systems in which uptake of radiolabeled drug and phosphorylation of drug by tumor cells are the endpoints deserves serious mention. MTX, 5-FU, 6-mercaptopurine, and ARA-C have each been studied and some clinical correlation with response of human acute leukemia to these agents demonstrated. However, Smyth et al,[38] found no correlation between uptake, deamination, or phosphorylation of ARA-C by leukemic blast cells and clinical response to a regimen containing that drug. Furthermore, Chang et al,[39] found no utility in the measurement of drug uptake or of intracellular activating enzymes for ARA-C or daunorubicin, or for measurements of the ratio of activating to degradative enzymes for ARA-C ("K/D ratio"), in predicting drug responsiveness of patients with acute leukemia. Test systems based on drug uptake and metabolism, it would appear, can hope at best to exclude ineffective agents, rather than to consistently select effective ones. In addition, some drugs are either unavailable in radioactive form or metabolized to cytotoxic moieties that may not contain the label.

2.5. Systems Based on Loss of Reproductive Integrity

Probably the most appealing approach, in theory at least, involves the application of in vitro testing procedures that quantitatively measure loss of reproductive integrity. This, of course, involves having cells grow in tissue culture. Unfortunately, human solid tumors have been notoriously difficult to adapt to tissue culture; Fjelde,[40] for instance, reported good growth in only 21 of 138 (15%) of tumors in which culture was attempted, and Ioachim[41] points out the almost universal lack of success with human breast cancer. When one does succeed in adapting a human tumor to long-term culture, this usually results in very different behavior of the cell population from what obtained in vivo, both with regard to the growth fraction (which tends to be much higher) and with regard to tumor antigenicity (usually reduced).

2.5.1. Cell Counts

Of more potential promise may be the use of short-term primary cultures in vitro, in which one might expect a greater similarity to the growth characteristics of the host tumor. Holmes and Little,[42] using mechanical techniques of cell dispersion and plating small cell numbers into fixed aliquots for microculture based on a crude viability assay, employed multiple washings with Hanks' solution, both before and after exposure of cells to drug-containing medium, in an attempt to remove all grossly nonviable cells and debris. They reported a 70% success rate in establishing primary cultures from 152 tumor specimens. After 24 hr in culture, multiple test microcultures were incubated with drug-containing solutions for 72 hr; then both control and test cultures were washed and trypsinized to obtain cell suspensions, from which aliquots were reseeded into microculture wells. The subcultures were harvested in 3–8 weeks, the period necessary to obtain sufficient cell growth for comparison of treated vs. control cell numbers. The authors considered a 40% difference between control and test cell population sizes at the time of harvest to represent significant drug effect, for reasons not fully discussed. In 13 cases from whom clinical correlation was available, 5 of 5 who had response *in vitro* also responded clinically. Only 1 of 8 nonresponders *in vitro* demonstrated clinical response (to chlorambucil, an agent that may not have been activated *in vitro*), for an overall correlation of 92%. In no case was an attempt made to influence the clinician's choice of drugs.

2.5.2. Colony-Forming ("Stem-Cell") Assay

Some authors have reported encouraging results with short-term primary cultures that involved growth directly on plastic culture flasks[43] or Petri dishes,[44] but the general experience with attempts to establish initial selective growth of human tumor cells was quite negative until the advent of soft-agar techniques. Culture techniques employing soft agar were successfully applied in the late 1960's to the study of murine hematopoiesis,[45,46] and subsequently they were adapted to grow normal human marrow cells.[47,48] As early as 1971, Park *et al*[49] had adapted this technique to growth of a murine myeloma, and in 1973, Ogawa *et al*[50] reported the value of a predictive assay system, based on drug effects on colony growth *in vitro*, for the mouse model. The use of soft agar in the base or "feeder" layer has at least one major advantage: it prevents attachment of fibroblasts to the surface of the vessel,[51] thus preventing early overgrowth by these stromal components of most tumors. The use of viscid medium, such as semisolid agar or methylcellulose,[52] in the overlayer or "plating" layer appears to facilitate relatively nonselective clonal growth; it "permits colony formation by biologically heterogeneous tumor stem cells because they are immediately immobilized . . . ."[53] This tends to minimize selection pressures that can rapidly lead *in vitro* to dominance by nonrepresentative subclones.

Although other investigators had reported some success in the cloning of pediatric solid tumors with two-layer agar culture,[54,55] it remained for Hamburger and Salmon to devise and describe the application of this technique to predictive assays for chemotherapy in man. Realizing that the presence in the media of certain stimulators is usually obligatory for the growth of granulopoietic and mouse myeloma cells,

Hamburger and co-workers added to their agar-culture feeder layer a "conditioning factor" derived from the spleen cells of mice given injections of mineral oil. In 1977, they reported successful growth of human myeloma, ovarian carcinoma, and certain other tumors in primary culture with the use of such "conditioned" medium. [56] Colonies were grown from 75% of 70 patients with multiple myeloma or related monoclonal disorders; the number of colonies that grew was proportional to the number of cells plated, suggesting their origin in a single clonogenic cell; and colonies plucked from the agar that were tested by a variety of morphological, histochemical, and functional criteria appeared to be myeloma cells. In ovarian carcinoma, 85% of 31 biopsy and effusion specimens formed tumor colonies *in vitro*, [57] with or without the presence of conditioning factor, so long as macrophages were present in the plating medium. [53]

In non-Hodgkin's lymphoma, Salmon's group achieved growth of lymphoid colonies from 11 of 18 bone marrows microscopically involved by tumor and 3 of 6 lymph nodes histologically involved by lymphocytic lymphoma. A variety of normal tissues sampled, including bone marrow and lymph nodes, did not produce colonies in their system, suggesting specificity for the growth of neoplastic cells.

In 1978, Salmon et al[58] reported successful use of their system to quantitate the differential sensitivity of human tumors to various anticancer agents. They performed 32 retrospective or prospective clinical correlations in 9 patients with myeloma and 9 with ovarian cancer. The patient was treated with standard chemotherapeutic agents singly, which were also tested *in vitro*. Each tumor was cultured using the stem-cell assay technique, with prior incubation of "treated" single-cell suspensions for 1 hr at various concentrations of drug. The data were expressed as number of colonies surviving vs. drug concentration. "Sensitivity" was defined as reduction by a specified degree in colony growth at concentration times time ($C \times T$) products that were felt to be pharmacologically achievable. In 8 cases of myeloma and in 3 cases of ovarian carcinoma, *in vitro* sensitivity corresponded with *in vivo* sensitivity, while in 1 case of myeloma it did not. *In vitro* resistance correlated with clinical resistance in all 5 comparisons in myeloma and all 15 in ovarian cancer.

Recently, Salmon et al.[59] reported an update of results with the tumor stem-cell assay. For a variety of tumors, 26 of 42 therapeutic trials with *in vitro* sensitivity demonstrated clinical response (62%), while 102 of 106 with *in vivo* resistance demonstrated this phenomenon *in vitro* (96%). Thus, the frequency of false positives, using a single cutoff point for *in vitro* sensitivity, appears to be fairly high (problem with specificity). On the other hand, the frequency of false negatives was very low (excellent sensitivity). From a clinical standpoint, the most important criterion for usefulness of an *in vitro* assay is that an active agent not be missed (good sensitivity), suggesting that this assay, if results are duplicated by others, may be clinically useful.

Von Hoff[60] and his group at the National Cancer Institute applied the basic stem-cell assay as reported by Salmon's group, but without the use of the mouse-derived conditioning factor, which, at least in the case of solid tumors, is not necessary for growth in primary culture. They also have demonstrated growth from a wide variety of tumors, including breast, lung, and colorectal primaries, and a number of sources, including ascites, pleural effusions, bone marrow, and solid tumor specimens.[61] They carried out marker studies showing that tumor cells were, in fact, producing their characteristic products *in vitro* (melanin in melanoma, carcinoembryonic antigen in colorectal cancer).[62] In their first 66 clinical correlations, Von Hoff and co-workers reported an overall accuracy of 100%: 5 of 5 true positives (sensitive *in vitro* and *in vivo*) and 61 of 61 true negatives (resistant *in vitro* and *in vivo*). Thus, their preliminary results also suggest potential clinical usefulness for the "stem-cell" assay, using a two-layer agar system.

3. Current Areas of Promise

3.1. Labeling-Index Perturbation

3.1.1. Exposure in Vivo Correlated with Effect in Vitro

It is known that most chemotherapeutic agents, even those that are classified as cell-cycle-nonspecific, are more effective at killing proliferating cells than nonproliferating cells. Thus, one would intuitively expect that effective therapy with any agent, regardless of its primary mechanism of action, should eventually produce a decrease in the fraction of cells synthesizing DNA, which in turn would be manifest as a decrease in thymidine uptake or labeling index. Agents that block the *de novo* pathway of thymidine biosynthesis, such as MTX or 5-FU, would be expected to produce an initial *increase* in thymidine uptake via the salvage pathway (if operative); however, with subsequent loss of reproductive integrity, a decrease in thymidine uptake would be expected here as well.

There is now a considerable body of experimental and clinical data that appears to validate these assumptions with respect to the effect of chemotherapy delivered *in vivo* on tumor-cell DNA synthesis measured *in vitro*. Briefly stated, effective chemotherapy produces marked and prolonged depression of DNA synthesis in sensitive tumors, sometimes after an initial period of "stimulation," as measured by thymidine uptake. Ineffective chemotherapy produces little or no effect.

Table I summarizes the results of 15 separate investigations carried out in experimental systems since 1964. Different methods were used to assay inhibition of DNA synthesis, including changes in specific activity of labeled DNA,[66-67] and alterations in fractional incorporation of tritiated thymidine,[75-76] as well as effects on the thymidine labeling index.[64-65] Despite this and the fact that different drugs and tumors were studied, several common features are apparent: (1) cell systems that are sensitive *in vivo* usually demonstrate maximum inhibition of DNA synthesis of more than 50% for 72 hr or more, with maximum effects evident at 48–96 hr in most responsive animal tumors; (2) bone marrow and normal gastrointestinal mucosa may show maximal suppression earlier, with rapid recovery; and (3) antimetabolites, as well as alkylating agents and antitumor antibiotics, eventually produce depression of thymidine uptake in sensitive systems, even if the *initial* effect of the drug is to stimulate thymidine uptake via suppression of the *de novo* pathway.[72-73]

Limited data available for human tumors also demonstrate depression of DNA synthesis as a characteristic of sensitive cells, presaging response after chemotherapy or radiation therapy delivered *in vivo*.

Sky-Peck[78] was the first to report that chemotherapy *in vivo* was followed by depression of DNA synthesis *in vitro*, comparing the results of pre- and posttreatment biopsy labeling indices. Livingston *et al.*[79] determined the thymidine labeling index before and after an initial course of chemotherapy in 63 patients (see Table II). In 16 who had a 2-fold or greater decrease in labeling index after therapy, 12 had objective tumor regression (10 complete or partial responses), and 3 others were not evaluable for response because of early death or prolonged delay in the second course of treatment. There were 47 patients in whom no such change occurred in the labeling index posttherapy: 45 had no response. The correlation between change in labeling index and response (or failure) was consistent, regardless of diagnosis, the type of chemotherapy employed, or the type of metastatic site sampled (19 nodules, 2 bone marrows, and 45 effusions). Similar data have now been provided by Tubiana and Malaise,[80] Breitenecker,[81] and Elequin *et al.*[82] showing that depression of the thymidine labeling index after radiation therapy is associated with favorable response and no depression with failure. Durie *et al.*[83] have observed persistent *depression* of thymidine uptake into tumor cells of myeloma patients who achieved remission, with a rise to baseline levels or higher that precedes or is concomitant with relapse, in contrast to earlier observations that re-

Table I
Treatment *in Vivo*: Effects on DNA Synthesis in Experimental Systems

Investigator(s) and reference	System studied	Drug assayed[a]	Maximum inhibition of DNA synthesis (%)	Time to maximum effect (hr)	Time to recovery
Tew and Taylor (1977)[63]	Rat bone marrow	CTX, 100 mg/kg (single dose)	70	24	By 72 hr
	Rat GI tract		60	24	By 72 hr
	Rat tumor (B[CRA15])		75	48	240 hr
Rosenoff et al. (1975)[64, 65]	Mouse bone marrow	CTX, 200 mg/kg (single dose)	59	12	By 48 hr
	Mouse GI tract		85	12	By 24 hr
	L1210 leukemia (sensitive)		93	72	7 days
Wheeler and Alexander (1964)[66]	Hamster plasmacytoma (sensitive)	CTX, 10 mg/kg (daily)	80	48	7 days
	Hamster plasmacytoma (resistant)	CTX, 10 mg/kg (daily)	40	72	By 48 hr
Wheeler and Alexander (1969)[67]	Hamster plasmacytoma (sensitive)	CTX, 10 mg/kg (single dose)	70–80	48	—
	Hamster plasmacytoma (resistant)[b]	CTX, 10 mg/kg (single dose)	0	—	—
Brereton et al. (1975)[68]	B16 melanoma (sensitive)	MeCCNU, 16 mg/kg	80	72	(Early) by 120 hr
	B16 melanoma (resistant)	MeCCNU, 16 mg/kg	55	24	By 48 hr
	Mouse bone marrow	MeCCNU, 16 mg/kg	50	24	By 24 hr
	Mouse GI tract	MeCCNU, 16 mg/kg	80	24	By 24 hr
Wheeler and Alexander (1974)[69]	Lewis lung carcinoma (sensitive)	MeCCNU	82	96	Prolonged

Reference	Tumor/tissue	Drug, dose			
Shapiro (1972)[70]	Murine glioma (sensitive)	CCNU, 60 mg/kg	65–70	24–48	Prolonged
Laurent et al. (1976)[71]	Murine ependymoblastoma				
	Minimal effect (2/12 CR)	CCNU, 2.5 mg/kg	30–40	—	Assayed only at 24 hr
	Optimal effect (5/12 CR)	CCNU, 10 mg/kg	40–70	—	Assayed only at 24 hr
Tew and Taylor (1977)[72]	Rat bone marrow	MTX, 5 mg/kg	40	48	60 yr
	GI mucosa (sensitive)	MTX, 5 mg/kg	90	12	(Early) by 24 hr
	Rat tumor (B[CRA15])	MTX, 5 mg/kg	50	72	72
	Rat tumor (more sensitive)	MTX, 14 mg/kg	52	72, 96	Prolonged
Myers et al. (1976)[73]	Mouse bone marrow	5-FU, 100 mg/kg	40	48	(Early) by 24 hr
	Mouse GI mucosa		50	24	By 48 hr
	P1534 tumor (sensitive)		92	72	Prolonged
Johnson et al. (1978)[74]	P388 leukemia (sensitive)	ADR, 10 mg/kg	99	24	48
	P388 leukemia (resistant)	ADR, 10 mg/kg	55	8	16 hr
Houghton and Taylor (1977)[75]	Lewis lung (sensitive)	CTX, 300 mg/kg	80	72	72 hr
Houghton et al. (1977)[76]	Human xenografts				
	Slight growth inhibition	CTX, 100 mg/kg	4–30	50	50–100 hr
	Marked growth inhibition	CTX, 200–300 mg/kg	52–97	50	250–670 hr
Hopkins et al. (1978)[77]	Hepatoma 3924A (modest growth inhibition)	ADR, 60 mg/m²	50	168	5 days

a(ADR) Adriamycin; (CCNU) 1-(2-chloroethyl)-3-cyclohexyl-1-nitrosourea; (CTX) cytoxan; (5-FU) 5-fluorouracil; (MeCCNU) 1-(2-chloroethyl)-3-(4-methylcyclohexyl)-1-nitrosourea; (MTX) methotrexate.

bTransient inhibition of growth by drug-resistant tumors was observed at doses higher than those shown. At these doses, both sensitive and "resistant" tumor demonstrated decreased synthesis after CTX.

Table II
Treatment *in Vivo*: Effects on DNA Synthesis and Clinical Response

Tumor type	Number of patients studied	Number with ↓ in LI% pre vs. post	Response Number with ↓ in LI%	Number with no ↓ in LI% pre vs. post	No response Number with no ↓ in LI%	Overall correlation
Breast carcinoma	18	6	6/6	12	10/12[a]	16/18
Melanoma	23	6	4/6	17	17/17	21/23
Other tumors	22	4	2/4[b]	18	18/18	20/22
TOTAL	63	16	12/16[c]	47	45/47	57/63 (90%)

[a] One patient restudied prior to completion of chemotherapy.
[b] Both responses 50% regression of measurable tumor.
[c] Three patients inevaluable for response.

ported an expansion of the growth fraction after successful chemotherapy.[84]

As a clinically useful predictor of response, the study of labeling index pre- and posttherapy has two serious drawbacks: (1) the tumor must be accessible to repeated biopsy and (2) the patient must be committed to a course of treatment before its effect can be evaluated. Several investigators have reported preliminary studies to test a more useful hypothesis (if correct): that drug therapy *in vitro* may predictably suppress DNA synthesis in sensitive cells.

3.1.2. Exposure in Vitro Correlated with Effect in Vitro

In addition to the work previously cited with chemotherapeutic agents, other investigators have reported that depression of DNA synthesis by hormones *in vitro* correlates with clinical response in patients with breast and endometrial cancer.[85,86] Zittoun et al.[29] used a test system in which drugs were directly added to leukemic cells, at concentrations that produced a 50% decrease in [^{14}C]thymidine incorporation of control nonleukemic marrows after 2 hr; *in vitro* depression of labeled thymidine incorporation was more marked in those who responded to therapy than in the nonresponders. The mean decrease in 16 responders was 52% compared to 24% in 26 nonresponders ($p = 0.01$). No difference was observed in depression of [^{3}H]uridine incorporation between responders and nonresponders. Lippmann et al.[87] found that when leukemic blasts from patients were incubated 18 hr with dexamethasone directly added *in vitro* [^{3}H]thymidine, ([^{3}H]-TdR) incorporation was significantly inhibited in glucocorticoid-sensitive cells, but not in glucocorticoid-resistant cells. Furthermore, the minimal concentration necessary to achieve this effect approximated that necessary to saturate steroid-binding-protein receptor sites. The glucocorticoid-resistant cells lacked such binding proteins.

Dosik et al.[88] recently reported the predictive value of a reduction in the S-phase fraction of leukemic cells, as measured by pulse cytophotometry, by *in vitro* drug exposure when this was correlated with clinical response to induction chemotherapy using the same agents.

Problems associated with direct addition of drugs in *in vitro* systems include the following: (1) the drug may not be present in its active form in the *in vitro* system and (2) the drug (or metabolite) concentration achievable *in vivo* may not be approximated under *in vitro* conditions, either through oversight or (commonly) lack of pharmacological data. An attempt to circumvent these difficulties involves the use of "treated plasma," defined as plasma obtained from the patient shortly after drug administration, at a time when pharmacological concentration of active metabolites may be nearly maximal. Such a technique has precedent in the use of various dilutions of host serum containing antibiotics to determine whether adequate bactericidal concentrations have been reached.[89] The determination of antineoplastic activity of treated sera, for the purpose of determining duration of antitumor effect after a single dose, also has precedence in experimental systems.[90] Dixon and Dulmadge,[91] Hunt and Pittillo,[92-93] Smith and Grady,[94] and Valeriote *et al.*[95] have demonstrated the biological activity of treated serum, obtained from animals receiving a variety of antineoplastic agents, in cell culture or bacteriological bioassay systems.

Burns *et al.*[96] measured [^{3}H]-TdR incorporation by scintillography of leukemic cells incubated with pretreatment (control) serum vs. serum from the same patient obtained after 2 days' therapy with ARA-C. The period of incubation with treated serum was 4 hr. All patients who had depression of thymidine uptake by 65% or more showed response, while depression by less than 50% was not associated with clinical response.

Work by a number of investigators with both direct drug addition and the use of serum or plasma containing drugs (or their metabolites) suggests that depression of the thymidine labeling index *in vitro* may be predictive of clinical response. Yet none of these assay systems has been adopted outside the author's own laboratory, and many have discontinued this work entirely. Two major reasons for lack of further development have been the heterogeneity of human tumor specimens, which makes approaches such as scintillation counting or pulse cytophotometry impractical for accurate application, and the variability of DNA-synthesis rates in tumor tissue, related to such factors as blood supply and degree of oxygenation, which creates the problem of obtaining a representative sample for *in vitro* testing. Until methods are developed for the physical separation of tumor from normal cells, methods based on morphology, such as autoradiography, will have to be employed to count the neoplastic cell denominator accurately. With regard to the problem of obtaining a representative sample, this is relatively easy to do with pleural effusions or tumors uniformly dispersed in bone marrow. But how can one obtain a "representative sample" of a primary tumor mass or nodule for autoradiography? Neither local injection of [^{3}H]-TdR into a tumor nodule, followed by biopsy[97] or needle aspiration,[98] nor *in vitro* determination of the uptake of [^{3}H]-TdR into tissue slices made from biopsied material[27] satisfies this requirement. (Counting as great a number of cross sections as possible, from one edge of the tumor to the other, will minimize problems from lack of tissue homogeneity; this, however, necessitates counting thousands of cells per specimen, and makes application to large numbers of samples impractical for most laboratories.) Preparation of a cell suspension from the tumor specimen as a whole was described by Coons et al.[99] as an alternative approach in the autoradiography of human tumors, and it possesses several major advantages: (1) the sampling error is minimized, since all portions of the tumor are equally well represented; (2) the cells are uniformly and consistently exposed to the isotope; and (3) the counting of a monocellular layer of clearly defined individual cells is technically much easier than counting sections. The method developed in our laboratory[100] is a modification of the cell-suspension technique initially described by Mavligit et al.[101] in which exposure time was shortened by the use of high-specific-activity [^{3}H]-TdR and the Hypaque–Ficoll gradient system was added to obtain a purified suspension of viable tumor cells. Additional virtues of the method include its rapidity and relative simplicity (as many as six specimens can be processed in a day by one technician); its close reproducibility, confirmed by examination of split-sample halves; and the fact that results obtained by this method are comparable to those obtained using in vivo techniques. Braunschweiger et al.[102] using the same basic method, have now confirmed that results obtained in vitro in the mouse C_3H mammary tumor system are identical to the results obtained with in vivo injection of [^{3}H]-TdR in the same system. The reproducibility of results was determined by analysis of the differences between labeling indices for duplicate sample halves, read blind by the same observer (R. L.) in 102 cases, counting 200 cells per slide.[100] The estimated variance of the log counts for halves of a split sample was 0.01 (as determined from analysis of variance). Thus, the standard deviation of the logarithms of the ratio of two such labeling indices was 0.141. A statistically significant ratio ($p \leq 0.05$) is therefore any ratio greater than or equal to 1.9, and one may expect with 95% confidence that variation in the labeling index within the same cell population will be by less than a factor of 1.9. Henceforth, in our laboratory, an "effect" was considered significant if it was 2-fold or greater. Durie and Salmon,[103] using a modification of this technique, also determined by analysis of duplicate samples that a 2-fold difference in labeling index was statistically significant.

Thirlwell et al.,[104] from our laboratory, reported preliminary results of an in vitro predictive assay system based on 24 hr incubation of tumor cells in autologous "treated" serum (obtained with 10 min of intravenous chemotherapy) vs. control serum. The tumor-cell labeling index was decreased significantly in 5 of 6 patients who subsequently developed clinical response, and no such decrease was observed in 9 nonresponders. However, subsequent experience in our laboratory revealed that 24 hr was not an adequate period of in vitro incubation to allow for maximal drug effects on DNA synthesis to be evident, and only 1 of the first 4 patients subsequently assayed had a response that was predicted by the 24 hr test (Livingston, unpublished data). This fact, plus the considerations relating to experience with animal tumors (see Table I), led us to prolong the duration of incubation prior to harvest of cell cultures for autoradiography, with removal of aliquots for labeling-index determination at 24, 48, 72, and 96 hr. We retained the basic scheme of 24 hr exposure to drug-containing plasma for "treated" cells. Cell suspensions of tumor or normal bone marrow were incubated with control media (supplemented Ham's F-10 or autologus pre-treatment plasma) and with autologous posttreatment plasma containing chemotherapeutic agents or their metabolites (treated plasma). Drug-specific effects on tumor-cell DNA synthesis, as measured by the thymidine labeling index, occurred in treated plasma in 9 of 9 courses where a response to chemotherapy occurred *in vivo*, compared to 2 of 8 in which there was no response *in vivo*. *In vitro* effects in treated suspensions of normal bone marrow were noted on myelocytes in 14 of 20 courses associated with leukopenia and 0 of 3 in which no leukopenia occurred. Overall, the labeling index was affected in 23 of 29 courses with associated biological effect (79%) vs. 2 of 11 courses without biological effect ($p = 0.0007$ by Fisher's Exact Test). In line with the experience of others in experimental tumors, we observed labeling-index effects that predicted for biological events only at 48 hr or more after exposure to drugs *in vitro*.[105,106]

Concurrent with our human experience over the past 2 years, we have examined the feasibility of the same assay system as a predictor of response in the 13762 rat adenocarcinoma,[107] originally derived from a mammary tumor of chemical carcinogenic origin.[108] The overall conclusion was essentially the same: In 6 experiments associated with antitumor effect (decrease in measured mean tumor size relative to baseline for treated animals, or more than 50% reduction in rate of growth relative to controls), 5 demonstrated significant associated depression of the mean labeling index at 48, 72, and 96 hr in treated vs. control cultures. In 8 experiments without *in vivo* antitumor effect, none demonstrated similar effects on the labeling index.

3.1.3. Advantages and Disadvantages

There are a number of advantages to predictive assays based on effects on DNA synthesis. These can be summarized as follows.

1. On the basis of limited available data, there appears to be strong empirical correlation with observed clinical results.

2. The approach is potentially applicable to all types of malignancy, including the leukemias, lymphomas, and as much as 50% of material derived from solid specimens that at present does not lend itself to clonogenic assay.[61]

3. Results are available within 5–7 days from the time of *in vivo* sampling, rather than 10–21 days or more for clonogenic assays.

4. The denominator of cells assayed as tumor is morphologically verifiable, an important advantage in dealing with the heterogenous cell populations that characterize most human tumors. With the use of Romanowsky-type stains such as the May–Grunwald Giemsa, individual cell detail is preserved and fixing artifact minimized. These stains have the additional virtue of compatibility with autoradiographic emulsions.

5. The technique is relatively simple. A trained technician can process as many as 6 fresh specimens a day, including setting up cultures for labeling index assay. Another technician can read the results on slides from another 4–6. Thus, in contrast to manual colony-counting procedures, the labeling-index technique is potentially practical for widespread clinical use, from a time and resource standpoint.

Unfortunately, the labeling-index assay has a number of problems, at least one of which limits its practical applicability. This is the fact that the reliability of a 2-fold change as a measure of "effect" applies only to specimens in the range of labeling index above 5%, at least when cell denominators in the practical range of 200–500 are considered (Livingston, unpublished observations). If the labeling index is as low as 1 or 0.5% (one labeled cell for every 100 or 200 cells counted), the difficulty with interpretations of changes in the labeled denominator becomes obvious. For many human solid-tumor specimens, labeling indices in this range are common.

Other problems include the following.

1. There may be identifiable tumor cells present in a sample, but too few to carry out a reliable labeling index (200 represents a minimum, with labeling index in the 5–15 range).

2. Some cells that label are probably not "stem" cells, with potential for indefinite replication, but may be destined for only a few more replications, and effectively represent a "dead-end" compartment within the tumor. It would be desirable to avoid the inclusion of this subpopulation in the denominator assayed for drug effect.

3. Changes in thymidine-pool size can theoretically occur, without necessarily implying a cytotoxic effect, as a result of a drug's inhibition of *de novo* thymidine synthesis (5-FU, MTX) or of effects on thymidine transport across the cell membrane. These might affect the labeling

index and produce a spurious indication of effect on DNA synthesis itself. Weisenthal *et al.*[109] have suggested that a variety of antineoplastic agents that exert effects on *de novo* synthesis of nucleotides may cause changes in the intracellular nucleotide-pool sizes, which could easily lead to false estimations of DNA synthesis rates based on thymidine incorporation. This is an argument with some validity, which must be seriously considered. It may not be very important from a clinical point of view, however, since (1) agents that affect *de novo* biosynthesis would always be expected to cause a decrease in endogenous pool size of the end product, and therefore "artifactual" effects on thymidine uptake should always be manifest as an increase (via the "salvage" pathway), rather than a decrease in thymidine uptake; and (2) the labeling index, depending as it does on an "all-or-none" phenomenon with respect to thymidine uptake, would be expected to be much less influenced by changes in thymidine-pool size than scintillation counting. This assumption is, in fact, often made in experimental cell-kinetics work, and is supported by Houghton's observations, in which both fractional thymidine incorporation and the labeling index appeared to be a more accurate measure of effects on DNA synthesis than measurement of specific-activity changes.[75,76]

4. It is often stated that changes in labeling index (and other measures of metabolic effects) are less reliable than colony formation as a parameter of cytotoxicity, based on the report of Roper and Drewinko,[21] in which cloning capability of a tissue culture line *in vitro* was set as the standard. For reasons to be discussed (see Section 3.2.2), this observation may not be valid, even in the system to which it was applied, and is more questionable still with respect to other settings, such as tumors growing *in vivo*.

3.2. Clonogenic ("Stem-Cell") Assay

The background and development of this system have been reviewed (see Section 2.5.2).

3.2.1. Advantages

The colony-count differential assay system, as reported to date from two laboratories, may be summarized as follows.

1. There is good empirical correlation with observed clinical outcome, with excellent sensitivity and moderate specificity.

2. If the stem-cell hypothesis is correct *and* the cells that grow in this system are actually those that are critical for self-renewal of the tumor population ("stem"), the denominator being assayed is the one of

clinical interest. This is suggested by the fact that the thymidine suicide index for colonies of ovarian cancer[57] or leukemic clusters[110] is very high, much higher than would be predicted from the observed labeling index in most such tumors. Such observations are compatible with the belief that the proliferative "core" of the tumor is being studied.

3. All types of solid tumors will grow in the system with an overall success rate of about 70%.[61] Special conditioning factors are not necessary, unlike the situation with hematopoietic tissues.

4. Fibroblast overgrowth is effectively prevented.

5. There is an obvious potential for drug screening, using this system against a "bank" of tumors grown in short-term culture.

3.2.2. Disadvantages

There are, however, a number of problems with this assay as it exists at present. These can be summarized as well.

1. Some solid tumors do not grow at all, and for others the plating efficiency is so low that the number of colonies per plate (preferably ≥ 100) necessary to discern cell kill reproducibly is not attained. In general, the plating efficiency is from 0.005 to 0.01%.[61]

2. Except for myeloma, hematopoietic malignancies do not grow in the system, and success with lymphomas has been less than satisfactory.[61]

3. The success rate on material from solid tumors (about 50%) is materially lower than that on material from other sources, such as ascites, effusion, or marrow.[61]

4. It requires from 10 to 21 days for colonies to develop in adequate numbers, depending on the tumor type (in general, shorter for solid tumors and longer for myeloma). Thus, the delay in beginning therapy for an individual patient, based on the assay results, might be as little as 10–14 days or as long as 3–4 weeks. In some life-threatening situations, it is difficult or impossible to postpone treatment for this long.

5. In a small but definite fraction of those cultures that do grow, recent observations (Elson, von Hoff, and Livingston, unpublished) indicate that the colonies are *not* homogeneous, but that some can be clearly identified morphologically as of "stromal" origin. Some appear lymphoid, others to be composed of macrophages, growing alongside obvious colonies of tumor cells. Thus, it appears that the assay system is not entirely specific for growth of tumor cells, confirming earlier observations by McAllister and Reed[54] of growth by material from a hyperplastic, benign lymph node in semisolid agar. The implications are obvious: if the efficacy of anticancer therapy is to be determined on the basis of a change in treated vs. control colony counts, and the reduction

observed is due to lympholytic rather than tumoricidal effects, a "false-positive" assay would result.

6. Although every effort is made to prepare single-cell suspensions, it is impossible to be certain that single cells are always plated; the dissociation of cell clumps with more than one clonogenic cell could, by itself, give misleading results.

7. Some evidence suggests that time should be allowed for cells to recover from potentially lethal damage after drug exposure, prior to plating. Twentyman[111] showed, for the EMT 6 mouse mammary tumor, that measurement of the surviving fractions (in colony culture) at short times after administration of cyclophosphamide indicated a much lower value than was compatible with the measured delay in tumor growth. Subsequently, he reported the same phenomenon for the nitrosoureas: for 1,3-bis (2-chloroethyl)-1-nitrosourea (BCNU) in this tumor system, very little delay in tumor growth was produced by high doses of the drug, "whereas the surviving fraction assayed 2 hours after drug administration may be as low as 10^{-4} for compatible drug doses."[112] He noted, over the first 48 hr after BCNU, that the measured clonogenic surviving fraction in small tumors showed a 50-to 100-fold increase, and ascribed the phenomenon to repair of potentially lethal damage when the tumor was allowed to remain in situ. These observations raise questions about the validity of clonogenic assay as a measure of antitumor effect in any system where transfer of drug-exposed cells is carried out immediately after exposure. For example, cells grown in culture in the frequently cited paper by Roper and Drewinko[21] were harvested immediately after exposure to such drugs as bleomycin and BCNU for colony-formation assay, while harvest after exposure was delayed for variable intervals in the other assay systems to which colony formation was compared as a standard. The authors concluded that colony formation was "the most reliable dose-dependent index of cell lethality" and that "tests that measure metabolic death grossly overestimate or underestimate killing activity . . . ." Unfortunately, there was no in vivo measure of response to which colony formation (or any of the other systems utilized) could be compared as a valid measure of antitumor effect. The possibility remains that colony formation itself, under these circumstances, may be misleading. Twentyman[112] has further demonstrated that plating out cells into fresh culture medium causes progression of nearly all of them (in the EMT 6 system) into and through DNA synthesis during the first 24 hr. He concludes: "Therefore it is perhaps not surprising that the fate of BCNU-treated cells is different if left alone in tumors for 24 hours, when many of them remain in G1–G0, than if made to replicate DNA at early times after alkylation."

8. The colony assay as practiced at present is very consuming of

time and resources in the laboratory. As von Hoff has observed, to set up one tumor in culture for assay of 10 potentially effective drugs (approximately 200 plates) requires about 14 hr. Another 20 hr will be required to count the number of colonies on all the plates (from a 200-plate experiment). Furthermore, "experimental data indicate that one observer must count the entire experiment to insure consistency in counting."[61] Even for assay of only 5 potentially effective drugs, the setup and counting time for a *single* experiment would be about 17 hr (or more than 2 days' work) for one person.

4. Design and Direction of Future Studies

4.1. Pharmacological Considerations Generally Applicable to *in Vitro* Testing

The assumption is often made that the best approach to anticancer drug testing *in vitro* is to take a given, pharmacologically achievable concentration of the agent and test this, plus concentrations that are 10-fold lower (or higher or both) for a fixed period of time against tumor cells. The period of time is often 1 hr, and a more sophisticated approach may be to manipulate the drug concentration during that period, such that the resultant $C \times T$ approximates that calculated to obtain *in vivo*.[58,61] There are problems with this approach that are potentially manifold.

1. Some drugs (e.g., cyclophosphamide, dacarbazine) are not active as the parent compound, but require metabolic activation to produce cytotoxic effects. They thus cannot be tested by direct addition *in vitro.*

2. Actual human pharmacology data for many antineoplastic drugs, particularly new agents that might be of great interest clinically in "refractory" patients, are often scanty or nonexistent.

3. The dose schedule for which $C \times T$ is calculated when human pharmacology *is* known may not be analogous to the dose schedule proposed for a patient.

4. $C \times T$ is not necessarily a constant, even for a single drug in a single cell-culture assay system.[113]

5. A period of 1 hr may be an unrealistically short period of incubation, especially for cycle-active drugs.

6. Plasma protein-binding, often a major factor for anticancer drugs, is not considered. This may be relevant to the observation of Salmon *et al.*[59] that "the drug $C \times T$ for *in vitro* sensitivity is generally a small fraction (e.g., 5%) of the clinically achievable $C \times T$."

Nonetheless, addition of drugs at varying concentrations directly to media containing tumor cells has the virtues of simplicity, general applicability, and (for clonogenic assay systems) encouraging empirical correlation with clinical response. Continued work with drug-containing ("treated") plasma seems to be indicated as well, since it has these real or potential assets: (1) it contains pharmacologically achievable levels of active metabolites as well as the parent compounds, which makes possible the testing of drugs such as cyclophosphamide; (2) a combination of agents may be readily assayed in a single test; and (3) factors such as plasma protein-binding are incorporated in the *in vitro* setting.

4.2. Future Directions

4.2.1. Automated Colony-Counting

This could make application of the clonogenic assay a practical reality, since it would greatly shorten the time required by manual methodologies for counting treated and control plates. It would not, however, shorten the "setup time" required for initial plating, which is still considerable. Work on such a counter is still in the developmental stages.

4.2.2. Better-Defined Specific Growth Requirements

If the plating efficiency of human tumor specimens could be increased to the range (about 0.03%) that is achievable for normal granulopoietic elements, grown in soft agar with the addition of colony-stimulating factors to the base or "feeding" layer,[114] many specimens that now permit inadequate growth for clonogenic differential assay could be tested. It can be hoped, but by no means assumed, that such growth-stimulating factors will be identified and can have general applications, at least to tumors of a given histological type.

4.2.3. Development of a "Hybrid" Assay System

Some of the most serious problems with the two most promising predictive assay systems could be circumvented or eliminated if they could be successfully combined into a "hybrid," and the strengths of each might be preserved. What is envisioned is a system in which tumor cells are plated on two-layer soft agar (or a modification of that system), and when cell growth appears maximal, the "stem cells" growing in this system are exposed to drugs, with effect on "control vs. "treated" populations measured as changes in the labeling index at various times after drug exposure. This could be correlated with results in the standard clonogenic assay, where feasible, and with clinical response.

Such a hybrid system would have the following advantages.

1. The labeling index would likely be high enough to permit accurate application of an assay system based on changes in DNA synthesis rate to all specimens that can be successfully cultured, even those with too few colonies for clonogenic assay by differential counting.

2. The cell population subjected to assay would be representative of the critical renewal or "stem"-cell population in the tumor, if the "stem"-cell hypothesis is correct.

3. The target-cell denominator would be morphologically verifiable, so that normal host cells could be confidently excluded.

4. Since colonies from most human solid tumors usually appear in 4–7 days, and the labeling-index assay requires about 5 days, results should be available in less than 2 weeks. For most patients, this degree of delay would be potentially acceptable, given demonstrated predictive capability for the test.

5. Although leukemias and lymphomas seldom permit sufficient growth to allow application of clonogenic assay based on changes in the number of colonies that grow out in treated vs. control cultures, the cluster or abortive colony formation that does occur might permit application of the labeling-index assay, if sufficient cell numbers could be obtained.

Recently, some progress has been made toward development of such a system (Elson, Livingston, Osborne, and von Hoff, unpublished observations). However, a number of technical problems will have to be solved for it to become a reality. It would then have to be verified for its predictive value.

4.2.4. Clinical Application of Other Techniques

In addition to the clonogenic and labeling-index assays that have been subjected to preliminary clinical correlation with encouraging results, there are some other promising approaches for which clinical correlation has not yet been presented. These include at least one *in vivo* technique, developed by Bogden *et al.*,[115] in which human xenografts are grown in the renal capsule of the immunodeficient mouse. This has the advantage over earlier xenograft techniques that changes related to drug effect can be measured much sooner, and with greater precision. The *in vitro* technique of alkaline elution developed by Kohn and co-workers (see Section 2.1.2) for the study of mechanisms of sensitivity and resistance in alkylating-agent therapy may have potential applicability to the human setting for the same group of drugs.

5. The Significance of Success

If any of these approaches develops practical applicability to the prediction of chemotherapy response in specific tumors, a variety of results would follow.

1. For patients with biopsiable advanced or recurrent cancer in whom chemotherapy is indicated, the assay would allow for selection of those agents (if any) for which intrinsic tumor-cell sensitivity exists and rejection of ineffective agents from which the patient could expect only toxic side effects.

2. For patients undergoing primary surgery with curative intent, but in whom there is a reasonable likelihood of relapse, assay of the sensitivity of the primary tumor may give a good indication of sensitivity of micrometastatic disease, making possible selection of the most effective agents for adjuvant therapy, or, if this is not elected, for treatment of relapse in the event of its occurrence.

3. Application of this technique to primary human tumor cultures could have profound impact on the methods by which drugs are currently chosen, both for extensive preclinical testing and for clinical trials. It is conceivable that activity against a significant proportion of primary cultures may, for a given type of human cancer, be much more predictive of eventual usefulness in that disease than activity in the murine experimental tumors on which reliance is currently placed.

6. References

1. B. C. Giovanella, J. S. Stehlin, Jr., L. J. Williams, L. Shih-Shun, and R. C. Shepard, Heterotransplantation of human cancers into nude mice, *Cancer* **42**, 2269–2281 (1978).
2. L. Kopper and C. G. Steel, The therapeutic response of three human tumor lines maintained in immune-suppressed mice, *Cancer Res.* **35**, 2704–2713 (1975).
3. A. E. Bogden, D. E. Kelton, W. R. Cobb, T. A. Gulkin, and R. K. Johnson, Effect of serial passage in nude athymic mice on the growth characteristics and chemotherapy responsiveness of 13762 and R3230AC mammary tumor xenografts, *Cancer Res.* **38**, 59–64 (1978).
4. M. Cline, *In vitro* test systems for anticancer drugs, *N. Engl. J. Med.* **208**, 955 (1969).
5. D. Ho, J. Whitecar, G. Bodey, and E. J. Freireich, L-Asparaginase requirement and the effect of L-asparaginase on the normal and leukemic bone marrow, *Cancer Res.* **30**, 466–477 (1970).

6. W. Hryniuk and J. Bertino, The treatment of leukemia with large doses of methotrexate and folinic acid: Clinicobiochemical correlates, *J. Clin. Invest.* **48**, 2140–2155 (1969).

7. W. Wolberg, Determinants of human tumor sensitivity to fluorinated pyrimidine chemotherapy, *Ann. Surg.* **166**, 609–623 (1967).

8. G. Hahn and H. Mandel, The roles of various biochemical effects produced by 5-fluorouracil in early growth inhibition of *Bacillus cereus*, *Biochem. Pharmacol.* **23**, 2689–2695 (1974).

9. M. McBurney and G. Whitmore, Mechanism of growth inhibition by methotrexate, *Cancer Res.* **35**, 586–590 (1975).

10. W. Ross, R. Ewig, and K. Kohn, Differences between melphalan and nitrogen mustard in the formation and removal of DNA cross-links, *Cancer Res.* **38**, 1502–1506 (1978).

11. L. Erickson, R. Osieka, and K. Kohn, Differential repair of 1-(2-chloroethyl)-3-(4-methylcyclohexyl)-1-nitrosourea-induced DNA damage in two human colon tumor cell lines, *Cancer Res.* **38**, 802–808 (1978).

12. C. Thomas, R. Osieka, and K. Kohn, DNA cross-linking by *in vivo* treatment with 1-(2-chloroethyl)-3-(4-methylcyclohexyl)-1-nitrosourea of sensitive and resistant human colon carcinoma xenografts in nude mice, *Cancer Res.* **38**, 2448–2454 (1978).

13. J. DiPaolo, Analysis of an individual chemotherapy assay system, *Natl. Cancer Inst. Monogr.* **34**, 240–245 (1972).

14. T. Kondo, Prediction of response of tumor and host to cancer chemotherapy, *Natl. Cancer Inst. Monogr.* **34**, 251–256 (1972).

15. W. Gewant and I. Goldenberg, Effect of drugs on carcinoma of the breast in tissue culture, *Surg. Gynecol. Obstet.* **135**, 81–84 (1972).

16. R. Waters and K. Hofer, The *in vivo* reproductive potential of density separated cells, *Exp. Cell Res.* **87**, 143–151 (1974).

17. J. M. Yuhas, R. E. Toya, and N. H. Pazmiño, Neuraminidase and cell viability: Failure to detect cytotoxic effects with dye exclusion techniques, *J. Natl. Cancer Inst.* **53**, 465–468 (1974).

18. H. Wigzell, Quantitative titrations of mouse H-2 antibodies using ^{51}Cr labeled target cells, *Transplantation* **3**, 423–431 (1965).

19. H. Goodman, A general method for the quantitation of immune cytolysis, *Nature* **190**, 269–270 (1961).

20. P. Ronai, The elution of ^{51}Cr from labeled leukocytes: A new theory, *Blood* **33**, 408–413 (1969).

21. P. Roper and B. Drewinko, Comparison of *in vitro* methods to determine drug-induced cell lethality, *Cancer Res.* **36**, 2182–2188 (1976).

22. M. Cline, Prediction of *in vivo* cytotoxicity of chemotherapeutic agents by their effect on malignant leukocytes *in vitro*, *Blood* **30**, 176–187 (1967).

23. K. Wayss, J. Mattern, and M. Volm, Correlation of *in vitro* testing and therapeutic results after cytostatic treatment of animal with transplanted tumors, *Arzneim.-Forsch.* **25**, 77–81 (1975).

24. M. Kaufman, *In vitro* testing of cyclophosphamide on tumors, *Naturwisschaften* **62**, 446–447 (1975).

25. I. J. Bickiss and I. W. Henderson, Biochemical studies on human tumors. II. *In vitro* estimation of individual tumor sensitivity to anticancer agents, *Cancer* **19**, 103–113 (1966).

26. W. Wolberg and R. Brown, Autoradiographic studies of *in vitro* incorporation of uridine and thymidine by human tumor tissue, *Cancer Res.* **22**, 1113–1119 (1962).

27. W. Wolberg, Biochemical approaches to prediction of response in solid tumors, *Natl. Cancer Inst. Monogr.* **34**, 189–195 (1972).

28. F. E. Knock, R. M. Galt, Y. T. Dester, and R. Sylvester, *In vitro* estimate of sensitivity of individual human tumors to antitumor agents, *Oncology* **30**, 1–22 (1974).

29. R. Zittoun, M. Bouchard, J. Gacquet-Davis, M. Percie-du-Sert, and J. Bousser, Prediction of the response to chemotherapy in acute leukemia, *Cancer* **35**, 507–513 (1975).

30. S. Penman, Ribonucleic acid metabolism in mammalian cells, *N. Engl. J. Med.* **276**, 502–511 (1967).

31. J. N. Lickiss, K. A. Cane, and A. G. Baikic, *In vitro* drug selection in antineoplastic chemotherapy, *Eur. J. Cancer* **10**, 809–814 (1974).

32. J. Hurley and L. Yount, Selection of anticancer drug for palliation using tissue culture sensitivity studies, *Am. J. Surg.* **109**, 39–42 (1965).

33. W. N. Hittelman and P. N. Rao, Predicting response in human leukemia, *Cancer Res.* **38**, 416–422 (1978).

34. D. Kessel, T. C. Hall, and D. Roberts, Mode of uptake of methotrexate by normal and leukemic human leukocytes *in vitro* and their relation to drug response, *Cancer Res.* **28**, 564–570 (1968).

35. D. Kessel and T. Hall, Retention of 6-mercaptopurine by intact cells as an index of drug response in human and murine leukemias, *Cancer Res.* **29**, 2116–2119 (1969).

36. D. Kessel, T. Hall, and D. Rosenthal, Uptake and phosphorylation of cytosine arabinoside by normal and leukemic blood cells *in vitro*, *Cancer Res.* **29**, 458–463 (1969).

37. D. Kessel, Relevance of *in vitro* tests for predicting responsiveness to antitumor agents, *Natl. Cancer Inst. Monogr.* **34**, 138–145 (1971).

38. J. F. Smyth, A. B. Robins, and C. L. Leese, The metabolism of cytosine arabinoside as a predictive test for clinical response to the drug in acute myeloid leukemia, *Eur. J. Cancer* **12**, 567–573 (1976).

39. P. Chang, P. Wiernik, N. Bachur, R. Stoller, and B. Chabner, Failure to predict response of acute non-lymphocytic leukemia (ANLL) using assays for deoxycytidine kinase, cytidine deaminase and daunorubicin reductase, *Proc. AACR-ASCO* **18**, 352 (1977).

40. A. Fjelde, Human tumor cells in tissue culture, *Cancer* **8**, 845 (1955).

41. H. Ioachim, Tissue culture of human tumors: Its use and prospects, *Pathol. Annu.* **5**, 217–256 (1970).

42. H. Holmes and J. Little, Tissue-culture microtest for predicting response of human cancer to chemotherapy, *Lancet* **2**, 985–9987 (1974).

43. G. M. Mavligit, P. B. Barsales, J. V. Gutterman, B. Mackay, and E. M. Hersh, A rapid method for establishing short-term primary cultures of human tumor cells from fresh tumor biopsies, *Proc. Soc. Exp. Biol. Med.* **150**, 597–601 (1975).

44. Y. Hirshaut, G. H. Weiss, and S. Perry, The use of long-term human leukocyte cell cultures as models for the study of antileukemic agents, *Cancer Res.* **29**, 1732–1740 (1969).

45. T. Bradley and D. Metcalf, The growth of mouse bone marrow cells *in vitro*, *Aust. J. Exp. Biol. Med. Sci.* **44**, 287–299 (1966).

46. D. Pluznik and L. Sachs, The cloning of normal "mast" cells in tissue culture, *J. Cell. Comp. Physiol.* **66**, 319–324 (1965).

47. J. Sena, E. McCulloch, and J. Till, Comparison of the colony forming ability of normal and leukemic human marrow cell culture, *Lancet* **2**, 597–598 (1967).

48. C. Brown and P. Carbone, *In vitro* growth of normal and leukemic human bone marrow, *J. Natl. Cancer Inst.* **46**, 989–1000 (1971).

49. C. Park, D. Bergsagel, and E. McCulloch, Mouse myeloma tumor stem cells: A primary cell culture assay, *J. Natl. Cancer Inst.* **46**, 411–422 (1971).

50. M. Ogawa, D. Bergsagel, and E. McCulloch, Chemotherapy of mouse myeloma: Quantitative cell culture predictive of response *in vivo*, *Blood* **41**, 7–12 (1973).
51. O. Costachel, L. Fadei, and E. Z. Badea, *Krebsforschung* **72**, 24–31 (1969).
52. R. N. Buick, T. H. Stanisic, S. E. Fry, S. E. Salmon, J. M. Trent, and P. Krasovich, Development of an agar-methyl cellulose clonogenic assay for cells in transitional cell carcinoma of the human bladder, *Cancer Res.* **39**, 5051–5059 (1979).
53. S. Salmon, Human tumor stem cells and adjuvant therapy of cancer, *Adjuvant Therapy of Cancer II* (S. Jones and S. Salmon, eds.), pp. 27–36, Grune & Stratton, New York (1979).
54. R. McAllister and G. Reed, Colony growth in agar of cells derived from neoplastic and non-neoplastic tissues of children, *Pediatr. Res.* **2**, 356–360 (1968).
55. A. Altman, F. Grussi, W. Reirden, and R. Bachner, Growth of rhabdomyosarcoma colonies from pleural fluid, *Cancer Res.* **35**, 1809–1814 (1975).
56. A. Hamburger and S. Salmon, Primary bioassay of human tumor stem cells, *Science* **197**, 461–464 (1977).
57. A. Hamburger, S. Salmon, M. Kim, J. Trent, B. Soehnlen, D. Alberts, and H. Schmidt, Direct cloning of human ovarian carcinoma cells in agar, *Cancer Res.* **38**, 3438–3444 (1978).
58. S. E. Salmon, A. W. Hamburger, B. Soehnlen, B. Durie, D. Alberts, and T. Moon, Quantitation of differential sensitivity of human-tumor stem cells to anticancer drugs, *N. Engl. J. Med.* **298**, 1321–1328 (1978).
59. S. Salmon, B. Soehnlen, B. Durie, D. Alberts, F. Meyskens, H. Chen, and T. Moon, Clinical correlations of drug sensitivity in tumor stem cell assay, *Proc. Am. Assoc. Cancer Res.* **20**, 340 (1979).
60. D. Von Hoff, Initial experience with stem cell assay, in: *Proceedings of the Human Tumor Colony Conference* (S. Salmon, ed.), Alan Liss, New York (in press) (1979).
61. D. Von Hoff, G. Johnson, and D. Glaubiger, Initial experience with the human tumor stem cell assay system: Potential and problems (submitted) (1980).
62. D. Von Hoff and G. Johnson, Secretion of tumor markers in the human tumor stem cell system, *Proc. Am. Assoc. Cancer Res.* **20**, 51 (1979).
63. K. D. Tew and D. M. Taylor, Studies with cyclophosphamide labeled with phosphorus-32: Nucleic acid alkylation and its effect on DNA synthesis in rat tumor and normal tissues, *J. Natl. Cancer Inst.* **58**, 1413–1419 (1977).
64. S. H. Rosenoff, F. Bostick, and R. C. Young, Recovery of normal hematopoietic tissue and tumor following chemotherapeutic injury from cyclophosphamide (CTX): Comparative analysis of biochemical and clinical techniques, *Blood* **45**, 465–475 (1975).
65. S. H. Rosenoff, J. M. Bull, and R. C. Young, The effect of chemotherapy on the kinetics and proliferative capacity of normal and tumorous tissue *in vivo*, *Blood* **45**, 107–117 (1975).
66. G. P. Wheeler and J. A. Alexander, Studies with mustards. VI. Effects of alkylating agents upon nucleic acid synthesis in bilaterally grown sensitive and resistant tumors, *Cancer Res.* **24**, 1338–1346 (1964).
67. G. P. Wheeler and J. A. Alexander, Effects of nitrogen mustard and cyclophosphamide upon the synthesis of DNA *in vivo* and in cell-line preparations, *Cancer Res.* **29**, 98–109 (1969).
68. H. D. Brereton, T. L. Bryant, and R. C. Young, Inhibition and recovery of DNA synthesis in host tissues and sensitive and resistant B16 melanomas after 1-(2-chloroethyl)-3-(trans-4-methylcyclohexyl)-1-predictor of therapeutic efficacy, *Cancer Res.* **35**, 2420–2425 (1975).
69. G. P. Wheeler and J. A. Alexander, Duration of inhibition of synthesis of DNA in

tumors and host tissues after single doses of nitrosoureas, *Cancer Res.* **34**, 1957–1964 (1974).

70. W. R. Shapiro, The effect of chemotherapeutic agents on the incorporation of DNA precursors by experimental brain tumors, *Cancer Res.* **32**, 2178–2185 (1972).

71. G. Laurent, G. Atassi, and J. Hildebrand, Potentiation of 1-(2-chloroethyl)-3-cyclo-hexyl-1-nitrosourea by amphotericin B in murine ependymoblastoma, *Cancer Res.* **36**, 4069–4073 (1976).

72. K. D. Tew and D. M. Taylor, The effect of methotrexate on the uptake of *de novo* and salvage precursors into the DNA of rat tumours and normal tissues, *Eur. J. Cancer* **13**, 279–289 (1977).

73. C. E. Myers, R. C. Young, and B. A. Chabner, Kinetic alterations induced by 5-fluorouracil in bone marrow, intestinal mucosa, and tumor, *Cancer Res* **36**, 1635 (1976).

74. R. K. Johnson, M. P. Chitnis, W. M. Embery, and A. Goldin, *In vivo* characteristics of resistance and cross-resistance of an adriamycin-resistant subline of P388 leukemia, *Cancer Treat. Rep.* **62**, 1535–1547 (1978).

75. P. J. Houghton and D. N. Taylor, Fractional incorporation of ^{3}H-thymidine and DNA specific activity as assays of inhibition of tumour growth, *Br. J. Cancer* **35**, 68–77 (1977).

76. P. J. Houghton, J. A. Houghton, and D. M. Taylor, Effects of cytotoxic agents on TdR incorporation and growth delay in human colonic tumour xenografts, *Br. J. Cancer* **36**, 206–214 (1977).

77. H. A. Hopkins, W. B. Looney, K. Teja, and A. S. Hobson, Response kinetics of host and experimental solid tumour after adriamycin, *Br. J. Cancer* **37**, 1006–1014 (1978).

78. H. Sky-Peck, Effects of chemotherapy on the incorporation of ^{3}H-thymidine into DNA of human neoplastic tissue, *Natl. Cancer Inst. Monogr.* **34**, 197–205 (1971).

79. R. B. Livingston, A. Sulkes, M. P. Thirwell, W. Murphy, and J. Hart, Cell kinetic parameters: Correlation with clinical response, in: *Growth Kinetics and Biochemical Regulation of Normal and Malignant Cells* (B. Drewinko and R. M. Humphrey, eds.), pp. 767–785, Williams and Wilkins, Baltimore (1977).

80. M. Tubiana and E. Malaise, Comparison of cell proliferation kinetics in human experimental tumors: Response in irradiation, *Cancer Treat. Rep.* **60**, 1887–1895 (1976).

81. G. Breitenecker, *Strahlentherapie* **150**(5), 487–492 (1975).

82. F. T. Elequin, F. M. Muggia, M. A. Ghossein, P. H. Ager, and V. Krishnaswamy, Correlation between *in vitro* labeling indices and tumor regression following radiotherapy, *Int. J. Radiat. Oncol. Biol. Phys.* **4**, 207–213 (1978).

83. B. Durie, S. Salmon, and D. Russell, Polyamines as markers of response and disease activity in cancer chemotherapy, *Cancer Res.* **37**, 214–221 (1977).

84. S. Salmon, Expansion of the growth fraction in multiple myeloma with alkylating agents, *Blood* **45**, 119–129 (1975).

85. N. Burstein and R. Carey, *In vitro* assay for human breast cancer hormone respon-siveness, *Oncology* **29**, 470–483 (1974).

86. S. Nordqvist, *In vitro* effects of progression of DNA synthesis in metastatic endome-trial carcinoma, *Gynecol. Oncol.* **2**, 415–429 (1974).

87. M. Lippmann, R. Halterman, B. Leventhal, S. Perry, and E. Thompson, Human acute lymphoblastic leukemic cells, *J. Clin. Invest.* **52**, 1715–1725 (1973).

88. G. Dosik, B. Barlogie, D. Johnston, D. Mellard, and E. Freireich, *In vitro* drug sen-sitivity test to predict clinical response in acute myeloblastic leukemia (submitted) (1980).

89. S. Dunlap, The serum dilution bactericidal test for antibiotic effectiveness, *Am. J. Med. Technol.* **31**, 69–74 (1965).

90. K. Kline, M. Gong, D. Tyrer, N. Mantel, and J. Vendetti, Duration of drug levels in mice as indicated by residual antileukemic efficacy, *Chemotherapy* **13**, 28–41 (1968).
91. G. Dixon and E. Dulmadge, Cell culture bioassay for vincristine sulfate in sera from mice, rats, dogs, and monkeys, *Cancer Res.* **29**, 1810–1813 (1969).
92. D. Hunt and R. Pittillo, Determination of certain antitumor agents in mouse blood by microbiologic assay, *Cancer Res.* **28**, 1095–1109 (1968).
93. R. Pittillo and D. Hunt, Cytosine arabinoside sensitivity in actinobolin-resistant *Streptococcus faecalis:* The basis of a utilitarian microbiological assay, *Proc. Soc. Exp. Biol. Med.* **124**, 636–640 (1967).
94. C. Smith and J. Grady, Blood and urine levels of antitumor agents determined with cell culture methods, *Cancer Res.* **25**, 241–245 (1965).
95. F. A. Valeriote, W. R. Bruce, and B. E. Meeker, Comparison of the sensitivity of normal hematopoietic and transplanted lymphoma colony-forming cells of mice to vinblastine administered *in vivo*, *J. Natl. Cancer Inst.* **36**, 21–27 (1966).
96. C. Burns, S. Armentout, and R. Stjernholm, Prediction of the response of patients with acute nonlymphocytic leukemia to cytosine arabinoside therapy, *Cancer Chemother. Rep.* **56**, 527–534 (1972).
97. R. Young and V. DeVita, Cell cycle characteristics of human solid tumor *in vivo*, *Cell Tissue Kinet.* **3**, 285–290 (1970).
98. F. Muggia and V. DeVita, *In vivo* tumor cell kinetic studies: Use of local thymidine injection followed by fine-needle aspiration, *J. Lab. Clin. Med.* **80**, 297–301 (1972).
99. H. Coons, A. Norman, and A. Nahum, *In vitro* measurements of human tumor growth, *Cancer* **19**, 1200–1204, (1966).
100. R. B. Livingston, U. Ambus, S. L. George, E. J. Freireich, and J. S. Hart, *In vitro* determination of thymidine-^{3}H labeling index in human solid tumors, *Cancer Res.* **34**, 1376–1380 (1974).
101. G. Mavligit, J. Gutterman, and E. Hersh, Separation of viable from non-viable tumor cells using Ficoll–Hypaque density solution, *Immunol. Commun.* **2**, 2463–2472 (1973).
102. P. Braunschweiger, P. Poulakos, and L. Schiffer, *In vitro* labeling and gold activation autoradiography for determination of labeling index and DNA synthesis time of solid tumors, *Cancer Res.* **36**, 1748–1753 (1976).
103. B. V. Durie and S. Salmon, High speed scintillation autoradiography, *Science* **190**, 1093–1095 (1975).
104. M. P. Thirlwell, R. B. Livingston, W. K. Murphy, and J. Hart, A rapid *in vitro* labeling index method for predicting response of human solid tumors to chemotherapy, *Cancer Res.* **36**, 3279–3283 (1976).
105. R. Livingston, Depression of thymidine labeling index *in vitro* predicts effects of chemotherapy in patients, *Proc. AACR-ASCO* **20**, 317 (1979).
106. R. Livingston, G. Titus, and L. Heilbrun, *In vitro* effects on DNA synthesis as a predictor of biologic effect from chemotherapy, *Cancer Res.* **40**, 2209–2219 (1980).
107. R. Livingston and P. Johnson, *In vitro* prediction of solid tumor response to chemotherapy, *Proc. Am. Assoc. Cancer Res.* **20**, 240 (1979); also unpublished data.
108. A. Segaloff, Hormones and breast cancer, *Recent Prog. Horm. Res.* **22**, 351–379 (1966).
109. L. Weisenthal, D. von Hoff, and M. Lippmann, *Semin. Oncol.* (1980) (in press).
110. H. Preisler and D. Shoham, Comparison of tritiated thymidine labeling and suicide indices in acute nonlymphocytic leukemia, *Cancer Res.* **38**, 3681–3684 (1978).
111. P. Twentyman, Sensitivity to cytotoxic agents of the EMT 6 tumor *in vivo*: Tumour volume vs. *in vitro* plating. 1. Cyclophosphamide, *Br. J. Cancer* **35**, 208–217 (1977).
112. P. Twentyman, Sensitivity to BCNU and CCNU of the EMT 6 tumor *in vivo* as determined by both tumor volume response and *in vitro* plating assay, *Cancer Res.* **38**, 2395–2400 (1978).

113. A. DiMarco, Adriamycin: Mode and mechanism of action, *Cancer Chemother. Rep. (Part 3)* **6**, 91–105 (1975).

114. M. Moore, N. Williams, and D. Metcalf, *In vitro* colony formation by normal and leukemic human hematopoietic cells: Characterization of the colony-forming cells, *J. Natl. Cancer Inst.* **50**, 603–623 (1973).

115. A. Bogden, A. Ward, T. Gulkin, H. Esber, and D. Kelton, Ranking the activity of chemotherapeutic agents against individual human tumors: Subrenal capsule assay, *Proc. Am. Assoc. Cancer Res.* **20**, 323 (1979).

2

Estrogen Receptor and Prognosis in Breast Cancer

C. K. OSBORNE, W. A. KNIGHT III, M. G. YOCHMOWITZ, and
W. L. McGUIRE

1. Introduction

Breast cancer is the most common cause of death from malignancy in American and western European women. Unfortunately, improvements in the treatment of this disease have been scarce since the turn of the century, when radical surgery for primary disease and endocrine therapy for advanced disease were first introduced by Halsted[1] and Beatson,[2] respectively. The overall survival of patients has not been dramatically changed since that time, and the prognosis remains grim, especially for women with metastatic disease or those with primary tumors invading the axillary lymph nodes even when all the clinically evident tumor can be resected and good local control obtained.[3] Despite the poor survival statistics, many physicians seemed reluctant to accept new biological concepts or to investigate new treatment approaches.

The 1970's, however, will be remembered as a decade of change and innovation in our understanding and treatment of breast cancer. Although it is still too early to know whether or not developments in the past ten years will have a significant impact on survival from breast cancer, early results are favorable and have generated cautious optimism among physicians and patients. Several developments either were born

C. K. OSBORNE, W. A. KNIGHT III, M. G. YOCHMOWITZ, and W. L. McGUIRE • Division of Oncology, Department of Medicine, University of Texas Health Science Center, San Antonio, Texas 78284.

or gained wide acceptance during the past decade (Table I). The most important of these from a treatment point of view are two: the concept that breast cancer is usually a systemic disease by the time it becomes clinically evident, accounting for the high failure rate of local modalities of treatment; and the discovery of the mechanisms by which steroid hormones interact with target cells. The former has led to the use of systemic agents as an adjunct to local–regional therapy in an attempt to control distant micrometastases; the latter has led directly to the discovery and use of the estrogen-receptor (ER) assay to predict tumor endocrine dependence. Although firm conclusions about the benefits of adjuvant chemotherapy await longer follow-up, it is clear that these two developments have revolutionized the physician's approach to the breast cancer patient.

The ER story is an enlightening example of how basic laboratory research can contribute directly to patient care. It had been recognized for many years that about one third of patients with advanced breast cancer had endocrine-dependent tumors that would regress with appropriate endocrine manipulation. Previous attempts using various clinical parameters to identify those patients with hormone-responsive tumors met with little success, although such factors as age, menopausal status, disease-free interval, sites of metastatic disease, or response to previous endocrine therapy were considered to have some relationship.[4] In the prechemotherapy era, treatment with hormone manipulation remained the only effective form of systemic therapy for advanced breast cancer even though only a minority of treated patients benefited. However, 10–15 years ago, effective cytotoxic drugs became available, producing remissions in one half to three fourths of patients and relegating endocrine therapy, with its inferior response rates, to a secondary position in the minds of some physicians. The need for an accurate

Table I
New Developments in Breast Cancer, 1970–1979

1. Relatively effective chemotherapy for advanced disease
2. Feasibility of early detection: mammography, breast self-examination
3. Concept that breast cancer is a systemic disease
4. Acceptable alternatives (surgical or radiotherapeutic or both) to the traditional radical mastectomy
5. Adjuvant systemic therapy to eradicate systemic micrometastases
6. Reconstructive surgery to improve cosmesis
7. Mass education of women; participation by the patient in treatment decisions
8. New types of endocrine therapy: antiestrogens and medical adrenalectomy
9. Understanding of the biochemical mechanisms of steroid-hormone action; discovery and use of estrogen receptor to plan therapy and as a prognostic factor

predictive index for tumor hormonal responsiveness was obvious. If physicians could select in advance those tumors not likely to respond to hormonal management, then patients could be spared the morbidity and time delay of ineffective treatments such as ovarian, pituitary, or adrenal ablation and considered for immediate chemotherapy. On the other hand, if hormone-dependent tumors could be recognized in advance, then endocrine treatment might be considered the appropriate choice. With the discovery that a protein (ER) present in all normal estrogen target cells is necessary for estrogenic activity, investigators asked whether some breast cancers might be sufficiently "differentiated" to retain not only ER but also their dependence on the hormonal milieu. The resulting proposal that measurement of ER itself might serve as a useful marker for tumor endocrine dependence has now been verified[5]; patients with ER-negative tumors rarely respond to endocrine therapy, whereas about 60% of patients with ER-positive tumors have an objective response. Patients with very high tumor ER content and those with tumor progesterone receptor have even higher response rates that approach 80%.[6,7] Thus, steroid-hormone-receptor assays have proven extremely helpful in identifying hormone-dependent tumors, enabling physicians to individualize therapy for patients with metastatic breast cancer, and opening doors for new treatment strategies.

Recent studies of ER in patients with primary breast cancer undergoing mastectomy suggest another important use for the assay. Patients with ER-positive tumors tend to have a lower recurrence rate and better survival than patients with ER-negative tumors, indicating that ER may be an important prognostic indicator. Intuitively, this is not surprising if one accepts the hypothesis that the presence of ER indicates a relative degree of "differentiation" of the tumor-cell population toward normal (nonmalignant). In this chapter, we will briefly review other prognostic factors in primary breast cancer, and then discuss the rationale and use of ER in this setting.

2. Factors That Influence Prognosis in Primary Breast Cancer

A panoply of clinical and histopathological variables have been touted as having prognostic significance in patients with primary breast cancer. Some of these are outlined in Table II. Unfortunately, there is some controversy regarding the prognostic importance of several of these factors, and there is a paucity of studies designed to prospectively evaluate whether each is an "independent" prognostic variable. This subject has recently been reviewed in detail.[7,9]

Table II
Prognostic Factors in Primary Breast Cancer

Variable	Relative prognosis	
	Good	Bad
Tumor histology	Medullary, tubular, mucinous, adenocystic	Infiltrating ductal NOS, invasive lobular
Histological grade	Grade 1 (low)	Grade 3 (high)
Nuclear grade	Grade 3 (well differentiated)	Grade 1 (poorly differentiated)
Encapsulation	Pseudocapsule, regular border	Infiltrative, irregular border
Tumor size	Small	Large
Lymphocyte infiltration	(?)	Present (?)
Stromal reaction	Fibrovascular (?)	Dense, collagenous (?)
Necrosis	None	Marked
Lymphatic and blood vessel invasion	None (?)	Present (?)
Sinus histiocytosis of regional lymph nodes	Present (?)	Absent (?)
Regional-node tumor involvement	None	Present

Nevertheless, there is no question that certain of these variables are associated with high risk for recurrence and poor patient survival, and taken as a whole several patterns emerge. First, it is clear that the extent of the local–regional tumor involvement is an important prognostic indicator. A large primary tumor or regional lymph node involvement implies a high risk for eventually developing recurrent disease after local modalities of treatment. [3] In fact, patients with axillary-lymph-node involvement should be viewed as having metastatic breast cancer, although it may be subclinical at the time of presentation. Nearly 9 of 10 patients with four or more positive nodes will relapse and die of disease within ten years after radical mastectomy. [3]

Second, several variables that are thought to be morphological markers of the degree of differentiation of the tumor may have prognostic significance. Tumors that morphologically and metabolically most closely resemble normal breast epithelium usually have a more indolent course and better prognosis; less differentiated tumors, on the other hand, tend to be more aggressive and are associated with poor patient survival. Thus, tumors with a histological appearance reminiscent of normal breast structures such as the tubular [10] or mucinous [11] subtypes have a more favorable prognosis than infiltrating ductal carcinoma not otherwise specified (NOS). Furthermore, tumors with less morphological atypia (low histological grade; high nuclear grade) have a better prognosis than more anaplastic tumors. [8,12,13] Tumor necrosis, which may be related to the more rapid growth rate of poorly differentiated tumors, may also be a bad prognostic feature. [8]

Finally, several variables thought to represent host-defense-reaction factors may be important, although opinions are less than unanimous. The degree of lymphoid infiltration in the primary tumor and alterations in the regional lymph nodes (particularly sinus histiocytosis) are both thought to represent manifestations of host defense and are considered by some to indicate a good prognosis. [8,9,14,15] On the other hand, others have failed to document a relationship between these factors and survival in breast cancer[8,16] or have found them, especially cell infiltration, to be bad prognostic factors, [8,16] and the relative importance of these factors compared to other variables has been questioned.[17]

Nevertheless, the malignant potential of the tumor, and thus prognosis, must be related to the innate biological characteristics of the tumor cell as well as the strength of the host defense systems. The lack of agreement among studies attempting to estimate these variables morphologically may simply reflect the limitations of these qualitative techniques. More recent studies using morphological and cell-kinetic techniques appear to confirm the more rapid rate of growth and worse prognosis inherent in poorly differentiated tumors. Furthermore, they demonstrate that the presence or absence of ER is closely correlated with these parameters, suggesting that ER may be a biochemical marker of the degree of tumor differentiation and malignant potential.

3. Rationale for Estrogen Receptor as a Prognostic Indicator

The presence of ER has now been shown to correlate with several of the pathological features directly or indirectly related to the degree of tumor differentiation. Fisher et al. [18] recently investigated the relationship between ER and a number of clinical and pathological parameters using sophisticated statistical analyses in a group of patients with primary breast cancer entered into several prospective studies of the National Surgical Adjuvant Breast Project. A direct correlation between ER and nuclear grade was observed. Tumors with poorly differentiated nuclei were much more likely to be ER-negative (58%) than tumors with well-differentiated nuclei (11%). Similarly, tumors with high histological grade were more frequently ER-negative. Furthermore, tumor necrosis and the lack of tumor elastosis, both bad prognostic factors, were associated with negative ER status.

These observations are confirmed by preliminary results from another study (in prep.), done in collaboration with Dr. Fisher, of a series of patients with primary breast cancer treated and followed in San Antonio. In addition, a prominent lymphoid-cell reaction, a bad prognostic factor,[8] was also associated with the lack of ER. A striking pattern was observed in this study: nearly all tumors (98%) with absent lymphoid-cell reaction, no necrosis, marked elastica, histological grade 1, and nuclear grade 3 were ER-positive. These data strongly suggest that ER is an excellent biochemical marker for tumor differentiation.

The rationale for the use of ER as a prognostic indicator is supported further by studies of breast-tumor-cell kinetics. The thymidine labeling index (TLI) is a measure of the proportion of cells engaged in DNA synthesis at a given point in time and thus is an index of the potential growth rate of the tumor. Meyer *et al.*[19] found a significant association between low TLI and the presence of ER, indicating that tumors with slower proliferative potential are more likely to be endocrine-dependent. In a later report,[20] they extend their observations to show that favorable prognostic features such as tubular or mucinous histological subtypes, absence of blood vessel or lymphatic invasion, and well-differentiated nuclei were all, like ER, more commonly associated with a low TLI. In a similar kinetic study, Silvistrini *et al.*[21] identified three distinct subgoups of women with breast cancer. Postmenopausal women with ER-positive tumors had the lowest proliferative activity; postmenopausal women with ER-negative tumors and premenopausal women with ER-positive tumors had an intermediate proliferative activity; and the highest proliferative activity included younger patients with ER-negative tumors. The tumor ER concentration was inversely correlated with tumor proliferative activity.

Table III
Relationship between Estrogen Receptor
and Known Prognostic Factors

Factors	ER-positive	ER-negative
Morphological		
Histological grade[a]	Low	High
Nuclear grade[b]	High	Low
Necrosis	Absent	Present
Elastica	Present	Absent
Cell reaction	Absent	Present
Kinetic		
TLI[c]	Low	High

[a]Low histological grade = well differentiated.
[b]High nuclear grade = well differentiated.
[c](TLI) [^{3}H]Thymidine labeling index.

In summary, there is convincing evidence (Table III) to suggest that the ER protein is directly correlated with the degree of differentiation and negatively correlated with the potential rate of growth of human breast cancer, providing a clear rationale for the use of ER as a prognostic indicator for time to recurrence and ultimate survival of women with this malignancy. In the following section, we will review the clinical studies that support the validity of this hypothesis.

4. Clinical Studies of Estrogen Receptor and Prognosis

The first evidence that ER might be a useful prognostic marker came from the study by Walt et al. [22] of women with advanced breast cancer who had had an ER assay performed either on their primary tumor or at the time of recurrence. None of the patients had previously been treated with systemic therapy. Two important observations suggested that the clinical aggressiveness of ER-positive and ER-negative tumors might be different. First, patients with ER-positive tumors were more likely to have bone or soft-tissue involvement as their dominant site of metastasis; in contrast, more life-threatening visceral involvement predominated with ER-negative tumors. Second, the median survival from the time the original breast tumor was noted was significantly shorter with ER-negative tumors (21 months) than with ER-positive tumors (46 months). Although this was a selected group of patients (all had recurrent breast cancer), the data suggested that inherent biological differences that could directly influence prognosis may exist between endocrine-dependent and-independent tumors.

In San Antonio, we were originally interested in measuring ER in primary breast tumors at the time of mastectomy in patients with clinically localized breast cancer in order to predict endocrine responsiveness later at the time of recurrence. During analysis of this data, an interesting trend became apparent: patients with ER-negative tumors recurred more frequently and had a shorter disease-free interval following mastectomy than patients with ER-positive tumors. In 1977, we reported an analysis of 145 patients with operable breast cancer treated by radical or modified radical mastectomy. [23] About one third of the patients also received postoperative irradiation or adjuvant systemic therapy. At a median follow-up of 18 months, the estimated recurrence for ER-negative tumors (34%) was more than twice that for ER-positive tumors (14%). Furthermore, this trend was independent of other potential prognostic factors such as age or menopausal status, size of the primary tumor, location of the primary in the breast, the pathological status of the axillary nodes, or treatment administered after mastectomy. The results were particularly striking in the poor-prognosis group of patients with four or more positive axillary nodes; an estimated 62% of patients with ER-negative tumors had recurred by 18 months compared to 27% of patients with ER-positive tumors.

These data suggest that patients with ER-positive primary breast cancer have a slower rate of recurrence than those with ER-negative tumors. However, the study is limited by small numbers of patients in certain subgroups, by short median follow-up, and by the fact that the patient population was heterogeneous with regard to the administration of systemic endocrine therapy or chemotherapy following surgery. Recently, we have updated the study with the inclusion of additional patients (288 total), the exclusion of patients who had received any systemic adjuvant therapy, and with a longer median follow-up (28 months). Again, the recurrence rate of the ER-negative group is significantly higher than that of the ER-positive group (Fig. 1). Of patients with ER-negative tumors, 35% have developed recurrent disease compared to 21% of ER-positive patients. Tumors with an ER content of more than 3 fmol/mg protein were considered positive. Similar patterns were noted when patients were grouped by axillary-node status (Figs. 2 and 3), indicating that the prognostic influence of the ER status is independent of this important variable. Recurrence data according to various other prognostic variables are summarized in Table IV. Regardless of the menopausal status, number of positive axillary lymph nodes, or location or size of the primary tumor, ER-negative tumors recur at a faster rate than ER-positive tumors.

This group of patients has now been followed sufficiently long to begin to examine the relationship between ER status and actual survival

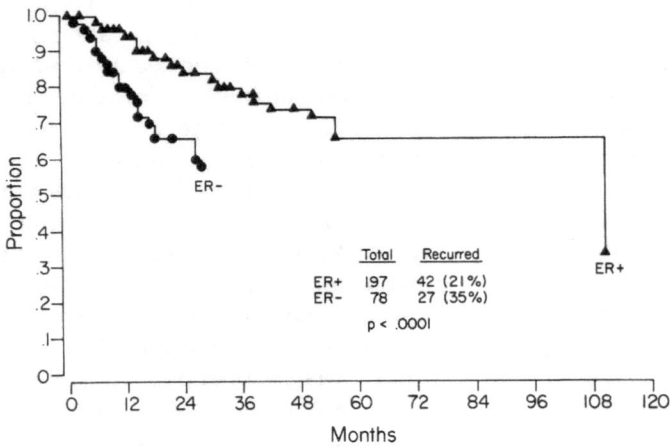

Fig. 1. Rate of recurrence for all patients as a function of ER status.

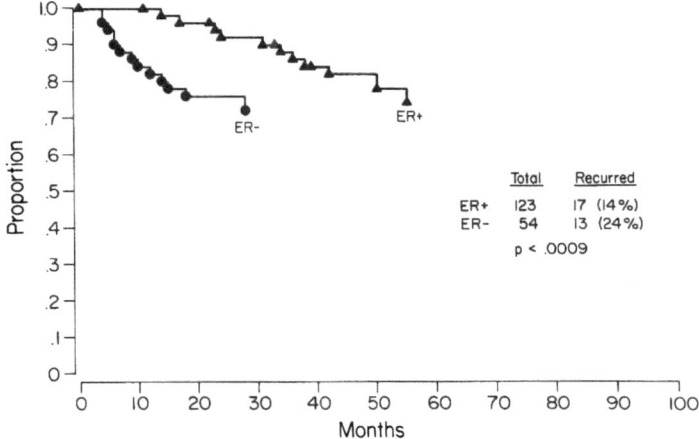

Fig. 2. Rate of recurrence for patients with negative axillary nodes as a function of ER status.

of patients. The cumulative survival of the entire population according to tumor ER status is shown in Fig. 4. Of 288 patients, 43 (15%) have died, including 22% of the 81 ER-negative patients compared to only 12% of the 207 ER-positive patients. More important, this difference in survival persists even when the patients are subdivided by nodal status (Figs. 5 and 6). Too few node-negative patients have died for the difference to reach statistical significance, but the trend is clear and suggests that the prognosis of these ER-negative patients may be much

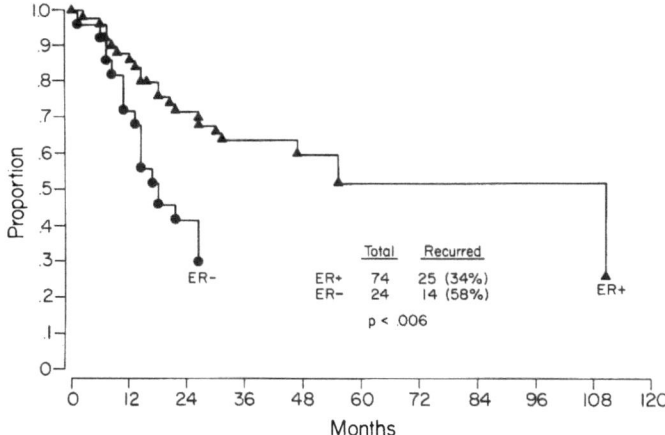

Fig. 3. Rate of recurrence for patients with positive axillary nodes as a function of ER status.

Table IV
Recurrence by Estrogen-Receptor Status
and Other Prognostic Variables

Patients and prognostic variables	Recurrence at 2 years (%)	
	ER+	ER −
Total patients	18	35
Menopausal status		
Pre	18	35
Post	15	38
Node status		
0	8	26
1–3	16	43
>3	40	68
Tumor location		
Outer	12	32
Inner plus central	12	50
Tumor size[a]		
2–5 cm	14	36

[a]There were too few small tumors (<2 cm) or large
tumors (> 5 cm) to draw firm conclusions.

worse than one might predict from the absence of lymph-node involvement. A dramatic difference in survival is noted in the node-positive
group. ER-positive, node-positive patients are currently dying at a rate
similar to that of the ER-negative, node-negative group. On the other
hand, nearly half the ER-negative, node-positive patients (43%) have

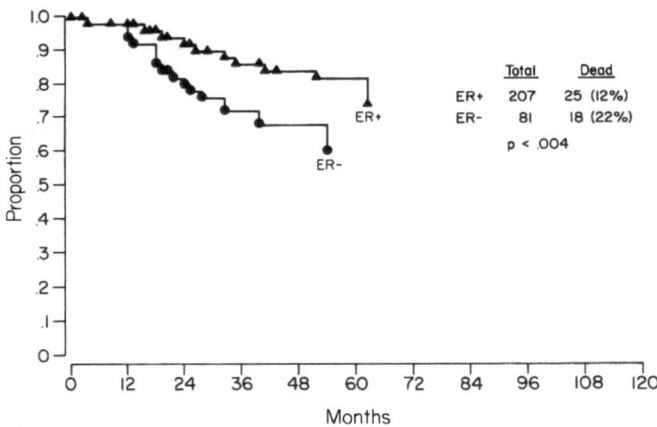

Fig. 4. Cumulative survial for all patients as a function of ER status.

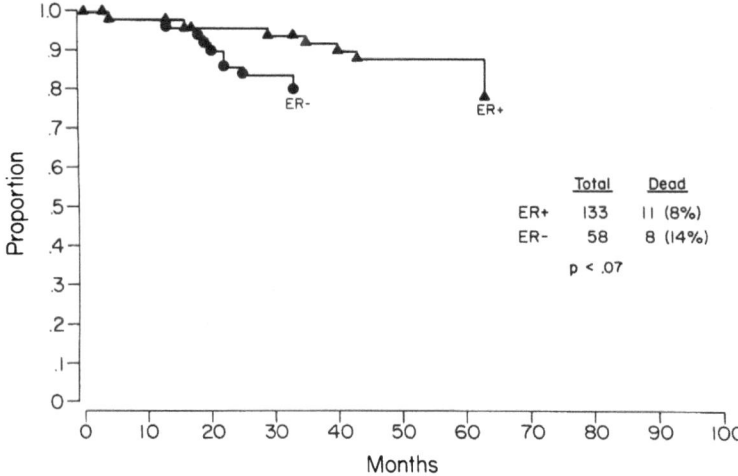

Fig. 5. Cumulative survival for patients with negative axillary nodes as a function of ER status.

already died despite a median follow-up after mastectomy of only slightly more than 2 years. The prognosis of this group of patients is indeed grave.

Thus, our studies indicate that the ER status of the primary breast tumor is an important independent prognostic variable for recurrence and survival of patients with this malignancy. Additional follow-up will be required to determine whether these patterns persist with time.

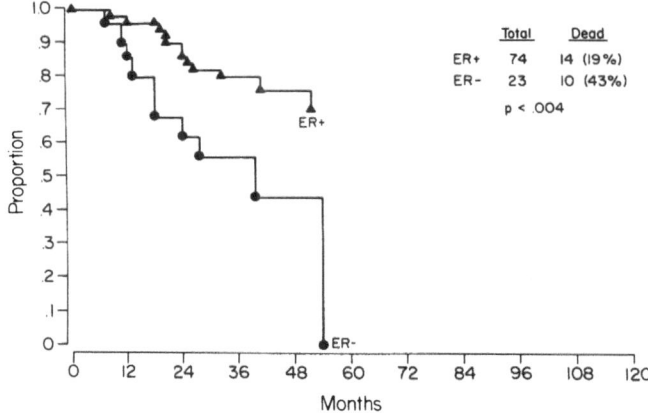

Fig. 6. Cumulative survival for patients with positive axillary nodes as a function of ER status.

Data from several other centers have now confirmed our results. Preliminary studies by DeSombre *et al.* [24] and Rich *et al.* [25] have found a shorter disease-free interval and more recurrences in ER-negative patients, though these studies do not address whether the effect of ER is independent of other variables. Allerga *et al.* [26] have reported a more thorough study and have found a relationship between ER status and disease-free interval that is strikingly similar to our own data. They measured recurrence rates on 292 women with breast cancer who had an ER assay either on the primary tumor or at the time of recurrence. They found prolonged disease-free survival in patients with ER-positive tumors that was independent of age, menopausal status, tumor size, or nodal status. Furthermore, the pattern persisted when patients who had an assay performed on a metastatic lesion only and those who had adjuvant therapy after mastectomy were excluded from analysis. These authors found no relationship between recurrence rates and the presence of receptors for progesterone, androgens, or glucocorticoids.

A series of reports [27-29] from the Tenovus Institute in Cardiff, Wales, and City Hospital in Nottingham, England, further supports the relationship among ER, tumor differentiation, and recurrence rates and survival of patients with breast cancer. ER-positive tumors were associated with better morphological differentiation, a longer disease-free interval after surgery, and longer survival than ER-negative tumors. However, several differences exist between these studies and those reported earlier. First, the prognostic value of ER was confined to the group of patients with positive lymph nodes and was not observed in node-negative patients. Second, although the data were not presented, the authors claimed that a relationship between ER status and prognosis could not be demonstrated in premenopausal patients. The explanation for these disparate results is not clear, but perhaps is related to differences in staging technique, method of ER assay, or differences in primary treatment, since simple mastectomy with node biopsy only was used in this study. The validity of these findings is suspect in light of a separate report from Great Britain co-authored by two of the investigators involved in the previous study showing that recurrence rates are significantly higher in patients with ER-negative tumors, a pattern that was observed in premenopausal as well as postmenopausal patients and in those with and without positive regional nodes. [30] In fact, the authors emphasize that node-negative, ER-negative patients are recurring at the same high rate as that of all node-positive patients.

Less aggressive disease was also found in patients with ER-positive tumors in an Australian study. [31] Although the differences in the number of recurrences in the ER-positive and -negative groups disappeared after 5 years of follow-up, patients with ER-positive tumors continue to show improved survival. A relatively poor prognosis for the ER-negative, node-negative group was also found in this study, suggesting that these patients are at high risk for recurrence even though the tumor appears to be confined to the breast at the time of operation.

In summary, morphological studies, cell-kinetic studies, and clinical studies from several institutions worldwide support the hypothesis that the presence of ER correlates well with the aggressiveness of the tumor and the prognosis for recurrence and survival of patients with primary breast cancer. The important therapeutic implications of these results are discussed in the next section.

5. Implications for Treatment

The data reviewed in the previous sections form the basis for a more rational approach to patients with primary breast cancer (Table V). ER-positive tumors tend to be well differentiated with a low proliferative potential and indolent clinical behavior. Thus, the risk for early recurrence after local therapy of these tumors is relatively low. ER-negative tumors, in contrast, tend to be poorly differentiated with a higher proliferative potential and aggressive clinical behavior. The risk for recurrence of these tumors is relatively high even when regional nodes are not involved with tumor. In addition, the majority of ER-positive tumors are endocrine-dependent and will respond to appropriate endocrine therapy, while ER-negative tumors rarely display endocrine dependence.

These factors have important therapeutic implications. First, since ER is an important independent prognostic indicator, clinical studies of new therapies for primary breast cancer should stratify patients by receptor status just as is done for nodal status, tumor size, and other prognostic variables. Second, knowledge of the ER status of a primary tumor opens doors to new rational treatment approaches by identifying

Table V
Summary of Estrogen Receptor in Primary Breast Cancer

Variables	ER+	ER −
Degree of differentiation	Well	Poorly
Proliferative potential	Low	High
Clinical behavior	Indolent	Aggressive
Risk for recurrence	Low	High
Endocrine-dependent	Yes	No

subsets of patients with different prognoses that may require different treatment strategies and also by identifying patients who may benefit from endocrine therapy as an adjuvant after local treatment.

Patients with primary breast cancer can be conveniently grouped according to the risk for recurrency by the status of the axillary nodes and ER status at the time of mastectomy (Table VI). Patients with negative axillary nodes and a positive ER assay on the primary tumor have the best prognosis and need not be subjected to aggressive adjuvant systemic therapy after mastectomy. Patients with negative nodes but also a negative ER assay, however, have a significant risk for recurrence that approximates that of node-positive, ER-positive patients as noted in several studies described earlier. Clinical trials of adjuvant chemotherapy should be undertaken in this group of patients on a research basis. Node-positive patients form a high-risk group. Those patients with ER-negative tumors have a very bad prognosis for early recurrence and poor survival and should be approached with intensive chemotherapy in an attempt to eradicate distant micrometastases. ER-positive patients with positive nodes are at high risk, but a variety of treatment strategies are of potential value. Since many of these tumors are hormone-dependent, endocrine therapy by itself or combined with chemotherapy deserves clinical trial, especially in postmenopausal women in whom the results of adjuvant chemotherapy have been disappointing.

The preliminary results of an ongoing clinical trial by Hubay *et al.*[32] demonstrate the potential usefulness of the ER assay in designing clinical trials. This study, involving patients with an ER assay on the primary tumor, compares standard cyclophosphamide, methotrexate, 5-fluorouracil (CMF) chemotherapy with CMF plus the antiestrogen tamoxifen with and without immunotherapy with bacillus calmette guerin. The first analysis of this study at 33 months follow-up is very interesting. The addition of tamoxifen to CMF significantly improves the relapse-free survival compared to CMF alone, an effect that, not surpris-

Table VI
Risk of Early Recurrence as a Function
of Node and Estrogen-Receptor Status

Axillary nodes	ER status	Risk
Negative	Positive	+
Negative	Negative	+ +
Positive	Positive	+ + +
Positive	Negative	+ + + +

ingly, is limited to ER-positive patients. Furthermore, as in the studies described earlier in which no adjuvant therapy was given, this study employing uniform adjuvant therapy demonstrated a better prognosis for ER-positive patients than for the ER-negative group. Immunotherapy has shown no benefit. Thus, adjuvant endocrine therapy with patients selected by the ER assay deserves further clinical trials.

6. Conclusion

The development of the ER assay to select hormone-dependent tumors and its use as an important prognostic factor for patients with both early and advanced breast cancer have dramatically altered our thinking and approach to this malignancy. It is clear that breast cancer is a very heterogeneous disease with a spectrum ranging from a slow-growing, indolent, chronic disease with morphology and biochemistry resembling those of normal breast epithelium to an aggressive, rapidly fatal illness with morphology and biochemistry suggesting a marked degree of dedifferentiation. As we learn more about the biology of breast cancer, we will be better able to subdivide patients into more uniform prognostic and treatment groups that will enable physicians to individualize and optimize therapy. The ER assay has been an important advance in this direction.

7. References

1. W. S. Halsted, The results of radical operations for the cure of carcinoma of the breast, *Ann. Surg.* **46**, 1–19 (1907).
2. G. T. Beatson, On treatment of inoperable cases of carcinoma of mamma: Suggestions for a new method of treatment with illustrative cases, *Lancet* **2**, 104–107 (1896).
3. B. Fisher, N. Slack, D. L. Katrych, and N. Wolmark, Ten year followup of breast cancer patients in a cooperative clinical trial evaluating surgical adjuvant chemotherapy, *Surg. Gynecol. Obstet.* **140**, 528–534 (1975).
4. B. A. Stoll, *Hormonal Management in Breast Cancer*, J. B. Lippincott, Philadelphia (1969).
5. W. L. McGuire, P. P. Carbone, and E. P. Vollmer, *Estrogen Receptors in Human Breast Cancer*, Raven Press, New York (1975).
6. C. K. Osborne and W. L. McGuire, in: *Breast Cancer*, Vol. 1 (B. Hoogstraten and R. McDivitt, eds.), CRC Press, West Palm Beach (1980) (in press).
7. K. B. Horwitz, W. L. McGuire, O. H. Pearson, and A. Segaloff, Predicting response to endocrine therapy in human breast cancer: A hypothesis, *Science* **189**, 726–727 (1975).
8. E. R. Fisher, Pathology of breast cancer, in: *Breast Cancer: Advances in Research and Treatment*, Vol. 1 (W. L. McGuire, ed.), pp. 43–123, Plenum Press, New York (1977).
9. M. R. Aldersan, I. Hamlin, and M. D. Staunton, The relative significance of prognostic factors in breast carcinoma, *Br. J. Cancer* **25**, 646–656 (1971).

10. H. B. Taylor and H. J. Norris, Well-differentiated carcinoma of the breast, *Cancer* **25**, 687–692 (1970).
11. H. J. Norris and H. B. Taylor, Prognosis of mucinous (gelatinous) carcinoma of the breast, *Cancer* **18**, 879–885 (1965).
12. H. J. G. Bloom, Prognosis in carcinoma of the breast, *Br. J. Cancer* **4**, 259–288 (1950).
13. H. R. Champion, I. W. Wallace, and R. J. Prescot, Histology in breast cancer prognosis, *Br. J. Cancer* **26**, 129–138 (1972).
14. M. M. Black, F. D. Speer, and S. R. Opler, Structural representations of tumor–host relationships in mammary carcinoma—biologic and prognostic significance, *Am. J. Clin. Pathol.* **26**, 250–265 (1956).
15. O. T. Anastassiades and D. M. Pryce, Immunological significance of the morphological change in lymph nodes draining breast cancer, *Br. J. Cancer* **20**, 239–249 (1966).
16. S. J. Kister, S. C. Sommers, C. D. Haagensen, G. H. Friedell, E. Cooley, and A. Varina, Nuclear grade and sinus histocytosis in cancer of the breast, *Cancer* **23**, 570–575 (1969).
17. S. G. Silverberg, G. R. Chitale, A. D. Hinel, A. B. Frazier, and S. H. Levitt, Sinus histiocytosis and mammary carcinoma—study of 366 radical mastectomies and a historical review, *Cancer* **26**, 1177–1185 (1970).
18. E. R. Fisher, C. K. Redmond, H. Lier, H. Rockette, and B. Fisher, Correlation of estrogen receptor and pathologic characteristics of invasive breast cancer, *Cancer* **45**, 349–353 (1980).
19. J. S. Meyer, B. R. Rao, S. C. Stevens, and W. L. White, Low incidence of estrogen receptor in breast carcinomas with rapid rates of cellular replication, *Cancer* **40**, 2290–2298 (1977).
20. J. S. Meyer, W. C. Bauer, and B. R. Rao, Subpopulations of breast carcinoma defined by S-phase fraction, morphology, and estrogen receptor content, *Lab Invest.* **39**, 225–235 (1978).
21. R. Silvestrini, M. G. Daidone, and G. DiFronzo, Relationship between proliferative activity and estrogen receptors in breast cancer, *Cancer* **44**, 665–670 (1979).
22. A. J. Walt, A. Singhakowinta, S. C. Brooks, and A. Cortez, The surgical implications of estrophile protein estimations in carcinoma of the breast, *Surgery* **80**, 506–512 (1976).
23. W. A. Knight, R. B. Livingston, E. J. Gregory, and W. L. McGuire, Estrogen receptor is an independent prognostic factor for early recurrence in breast cancer, *Cancer Res.* **37**, 4669–4671 (1977).
24. E. R. DeSombre, G. L. Greene, and E. V. Jensen, Estrophilin and endocrine responsiveness of breast cancer, in: *Hormones, Receptors, and Breast Cancer* (W. L. McGuire, ed.), pp. 1–14, Raven Press, New York (1978).
25. M. A. Rich, P. Furmanski, and S. C. Brooks, Prognostic value of estrogen receptor determinations in patients with breast cancer, *Cancer Res.* **38**, 4296–4298 (1978).
26. J. C. Allegra, M. E. Lippman, R. Simon, E. B. Thompson, A. Barlock, L. Green, K. K. Huff, H. M. T. Do, S. C. Aitken, and R. Warren, Association between steroid hormone receptor status and disease-free interval in breast cancer, *Cancer Treat. Rep.* **63**, 1271–1277 (1979).
27. P. V. Maynard, R. W. Blamey, C. W. Elston, J. L. Haybittle, and K. Griffiths, Estrogen receptor assay in primary breast cancer and early recurrence of the disease, *Cancer Res.* **38**, 4292–4295 (1978).
28. P. V. Maynard, C. J. Davies, R. W. Blamey, C. W. Elston, J. Johnson, and K. Griffiths, Relationship between oestrogen-receptor content and histological grade in human primary breast tumors, *Br. J. Cancer* **38**, 745–748 (1978).

29. H. M. Bishop, C. W. Elston, R. W. Blamey, J. L. Haybittle, R. I. Nicholson, and K. Griffiths, Relationship of oestrogen-receptor status to survival in breast cancer, *Lancet* **2**, 283–284 (1979).
30. T. Cooke, R. Shields, D. George, P. Maynard, and K. Griffiths, Oestrogen receptors and prognosis in early breast cancer, *Lancet* **1**, 995–997 (1979).
31. R. Hahnel, T. Woodings, and A. B. Vivan, Prognostic value of estrogen receptors in primary breast cancer, *Cancer* **44**, 671–675 (1979).
32. C. A. Hubay, O. H. Pearson, J. S. Marshall, R. S. Rhodes, S. M. Debanne, E. G. Mansour, R. E. Hermann, J. C. Jones, W. J. Flynn, C. Eckert, and W. L. McGuire, Antiestrogen, cytotoxic chemotherapy, and BCG vaccination in stage II breast cancer, *Surgery,* **87**, 494–501 (1980).

3

Benign Breast Disease

PIERRE MAUVAIS-JARVIS, REGINE SITRUK-WARE, and
FREDERIQUE KUTTENN

1. Introduction

There are many discrepancies in the definition of benign breast disease. For most physicians, this disease is essentially defined by the observation of masses in the breast that remain permanent throughout the menstrual cycle. For the radiologist, the diagnosis of benign breast disease is complemented by the visualization of abnormalities in breast transparence by mammography. For pathologists, benign breast disease should be classified only from a morphological point of view. Their classifications of different forms of the disease are based on the microscopic evaluation of objective cellular abnormalities occurring in a given anatomical site of the mammary gland.

Until recent years, and this remains true for many specialists in the mammary gland, the definition of benign breast disease was often restricted to chronic fibrocystic disease. In addition, epidemiological studies concerning the relationship between benign breat disease and mammary carcinoma have been essentially carried out from retrospective inquiries of women with prior breast biopsy. In fact, this attitude seems very restrictive. It is indeed undisputed that many women with breast cancer do not give histories of benign mastopathy, but it should be pointed out that until recently, the practice of systematic breast examination during the reproductive years has not been widespread. There-

PIERRE MAUVAIS-JARVIS, REGINE SITRUK-WARE, and FREDERIQUE KUT-
TENN • Department of Reproductive Endocrinology, Hôpital Necker, 75730 Paris Cedex
15, France.

fore, it is likely that many women in whom mammary cancer is found actually had previous benign lesions that were never diagnosed because they had never been looked for or because of the difficulties encountered in establishing the definition and the limits of the disease.

However, benign breast disease may be considered, for different reasons, as an important evolutional link between the normal mammary gland and the carcinoma.

If one accepts that the tumor doubling time of mammary carcinoma is, on the average, 100 days, it follows that a clinically detectable tumor 2 cm in diameter has already been growing for a period of 9–10 years. That would comprise 100–130 menstrual cycles. This underlines the importance of the study and treatment of breast lesions during a woman's reproductive years.

In addition, structural studies using the electron microscope and immunological studies[1] indicate a continuum going from fibrocystic disease to invasive carcinoma, passing through carcinoma *in situ*. Patients with fibrocystic lesions constitute a population with a higher than normal risk of cancer, evaluated by various authors as being from 2 to 5 times that of normal women. [2-4]

The previous finding of the presence of specific receptors for estradiol and progesterone in breast cancer, in benign breast disease, and its postulation in the normal breast[5] definitely classified the mammary gland as hormone-dependent.

In addition, there are now many studies that suggest that sex hormones (in particular estrogen and progesterone derivatives) can modify the frequency of benign breast diseases and their transformation into carcinoma. Thus, from an endocrinological point of view, it does not seem reasonable to consider benign breast disease only as a restrictive entity limited to histological and mammographic characteristics; it is now more appropriate to have an overall view of this disease in terms of hormone dependency and of hormonal milieu permitting the development of breast lesions with different steps of cellular alterations.

2. Histopathology of Benign Breast Disease

2.1. Structure of the Normal Mammary Gland

The normal breast gland consists of an epithelial parenchyma of acini and ducts, included in muscular and fascial elements, and of varying amounts of fat, blood vessels, nerves, and lymphatics.

2.1.1. *Epithelial Structures*

The epithelial structures are divided into 20 or more lobes, each emptying into a separate excretory duct terminating in the nipple. These lobes are divided into numerous *lobules*, each made up of 10–100 or more acini grouped around a collecting duct.[3]

The different collecting ducts join together to form the main excretory duct. These ducts might be divided into three different groups according to their size[6,7] (Fig. 1): (1) intralobular ducts or initial collecting ducts; (2) extralobular terminal ducts; and (3) main excretory ducts. [6,7] The lobules realize the basic structural unit of the mammary gland. Their number and size vary, and they are largest and most numerous in the young woman's breast.

The epithelial elements and the connective tissue are extremely intermingled. Thus, the morphology of benign breast diseases depends on the size and on the type of these different elements taking part in benign proliferations.

a. Acini. The acini consist of two layers of cells. They are lined by an internal layer of cuboidal or cylindrical epithelial cells, and a second layer is found around the base of the acinus. These cells are called basal

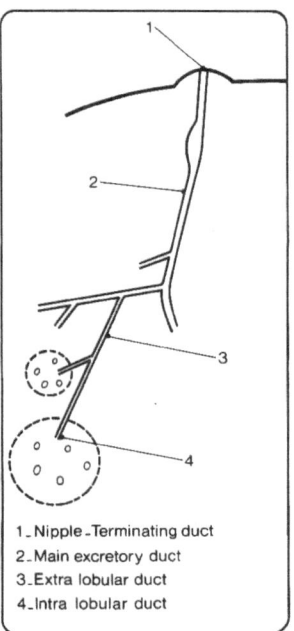

Fig. 1. Pathophysiology of benign breast disease. Organization of the galactophoric system in the normal adult woman showing areas where the different benign breast diseases originate: (1) nipple–terminating duct; (2) main excretory duct (mammary duct ectasia, hyperplastic duct, duct papilloma); (3) extralobular duct (cysts, fibrocystic disease); (4) intralobular duct (adenosis, sclerosing adenosis, adenofibroma).

1_ Nipple _Terminating duct
2_ Main excretory duct
3_ Extra lobular duct
4_ Intra lobular duct

cells or myoepithelial cells. Each acinus is enveloped by a fine basement membrane extending to the collecting ducts.

The lobule as a whole is enclosed by a thicker collagen envelope.

b. Myoepithelial Cells. These cells lie directly on the basement membrane and are considered as basal cells "in reserve" that will replace the secreting cells. They resemble smooth muscle cells and provide a muscular mechanism for ejecting milk from acini and ducts controlled by hormonal factors.[3] These cells have a special interest because their hyperplasia leads to certain benign proliferations.

The sex hormones, especially estrogens, stimulate the glandular epithelium to proliferate.[8] The epithelium becomes multilayered, the epithelial cells differentiate more than normally, and the cells change in that the nuclei enlarge, chromatin increases, and large nucleoli and mitoses emerge.[8] This epithelial proliferation, with cell change, is observed for example in estrogen-induced gynecomastia.[8]

2.1.2. Connective Tissue

The connective tissue consists of two parts.

After puberty, the mesenchymal portions of the mammary gland differentiate into an intralobular connective tissue, called "mantle tissue."[3] This tissue is concerned with the hormonal stimulation. A different collagenous connective tissue surrounds the lobules and acts as a supportive tissue.

In some benign breast diseases, multiple histopathological changes of structure occur in connective tissue, which exhibits a secretion of fluid, edematous, mucoid swellings of this stroma, and hyalinization.

The deposits of fluid observed in fibrocystic disease contain albumin thought to derive from permeable blood vessels and seem to be of great importance in mastopathy.[8] Histochemical studies in rats have demonstrated a rise of mucopolysaccharide content in the connective tissue after estrogen treatment.[8] Progesterone, on the other hand, inhibited the mesenchymal action of estrogen.[9] These deposits seem to be of importance for the fibrosing of glands and for the pathology of the human mammary gland in hormonally induced dysplasias.[8]

2.2. Pathology of Benign Breast Disease

The different benign breast diseases can be classified in different manners, and various descriptions are reported according to the different authors.

A topographical study of the galactophoretic system enables better understanding and interpretation of the most common lesions.[6]

2.2.1. Benign Neoplasms Originating from the Main Excretory Ducts (Fig. 1)

   a. Mammary Duct Ectasia. This is a common disease of the aging breast that frequently escapes detection.
   It begins with dilatation of the terminal collecting ducts beneath the nipple and areola. When present, the clinical signs are a tumor, or a nipple discharge either spontaneous or produced by a gentle pressure. The discharge may be serous, bloodstained, or more viscous.
   On gross pathology, the majority of the terminal ducts are involved and dilated. The duct walls are thickened by fibrosis and inflammatory infiltration of lymphocytes. Atrophy and fibrosis of the epithelium seem to be the rule, rather than proliferation. Fibrosis may induce retraction of the nipple. The duct walls are distended by an intraluminal material characterized by amorphous substance and lipidic crystalline bodies. These substances provoke an inflammatory reaction with sometimes a great concentration of plasma cells. Thus, this lesion has been called "plasma cell mastitis" by some pathologists. Papillomas are not found in mammary duct ectasia.[3]
   In some patients with duct ectasia, episodes of acute inflammation occur with enlarged axillary lymph nodes. Sometimes the ectatic ducts calcify.
   b. Hyperplastic Duct. The hyperplastic duct is a rare lesion. The ducts are focally lined by hyperplastic cells or filled by these cells. Some of the cells show variable degrees of anaplasia with papillary proliferations. These proliferations can form a *duct papilloma* located within the duct proximal to terminal, with a low grade of epithelial anaplasia. [6,7] However, it is often difficult to differentiate this lesion from a duct carcinoma.

2.2.2. Benign Lesions Originating from Extralobular Ducts

   a. Cysts. The more common lesions observed at this level are cysts. The morphology of these cysts depends on the diameter of the duct concerned. The cystic disease seems to be the result of the obstruction of the ducts by the edematous, then sclerous, connective tissue. Second, the duct is dilated above the obstruction.[6] However, since there is no microscopic evidence that obstruction of the ducts plays any role in the origin of the microcysts, it seemed likely to Haagensen[3] that the larger cysts originate from the microscopic ones.
   A solitary cyst is unusual, and more often a larger cyst is surrounded by a number of small cysts in the immediately adjacent mammary tissue.
   The wall of the cyst consists of a single layer of flattened to cuboidal

epithelium. The fluid they contain looks like blood-serum in recent cysts or is more dark-colored in old cysts.

b. Other Microscopic Features Frequently Found Together with Grossly Visible Cysts. The proliferation of duct epithelium is often observed and may fill up the lumens of the dilated ducts. But the proliferating cells maintain the characteristics of benign cells, and in the view of Haagensen,[3] this kind of epithelial proliferation does not predispose to the development of carcinoma.

Sometimes the intraductal proliferations exhibit a papillary pattern, but this must be distinguished from the intraductal papilloma developed in the proximal ducts.

The normal cuboidal epithelium of the ducts can sometimes exhibit *apocrine metaplasia.* The epithelium becomes columnar with large cells with small regular nuclei and abundant eosinophilic cytoplasm.

Speert[10] produced apocrine metaplasia of the breast epithelium in the rhesus monkey by administration of very large doses of estrogen.

Adenosis and *fibrosis* are also encountered in cystic disease. Adenosis consists of the benign proliferation of acini and ducts in a lobular pattern and is also called lobular hyperplasia. Usually it develops in small foci surrounding the cysts, but can acquire an infiltrative character and thereby become confused with carcinoma.

Finally, proliferation of fibroblasts in the breast stroma is usual in cystic disease.

2.2.3. Benign Lesions Originating from the Intralobular Ducts and Ductules

Three particular entities are encountered: adenosis, sclerosing adenosis, and adenofibromas. These three types of lesions originate from the lobules and the intralobular ducts.

a. Adenosis. The acini of the gland fields and to a lesser extent the small ducts proliferate, invade the breast stroma, and finally can stimulate fibrosis and constitute sclerosing adenosis.

When the proliferation is limited to small foci, it constitutes one of the features of cystic disease. But when adenosis grows as a pure type of epithelial proliferation, it leads to a palpable tumor called adenosis tumor.[3] Sometimes these tumors are clinically indistinguishable from carcinoma.

The adenosis tumor is observed during the menstrual phase of life, and some of these tumors have developed in young patients using exogenous estrogens.[3]

b. Sclerosing Adenosis. This is a variety of adenosis. The multiplication of the small ducts is surrounded by a proliferation of myoepithelial cells that secrete collagen, leading to fibrosis.

c. Adenofibroma. This is a frequent tumor that usually develops during youth. It is considered as the third most common tumor of the breast in present-day American women, after carcinoma and cystic disease.[3] These tumors are frequently observed after estrogen treatment and also respond to a growth stimulus during pregnancy, suggesting that their origin is in some way associated with estrogenic stimulation.[3]

The gross appearance of adenofibroma is characteristic. It is sharply delimited from the surrounding tissue.

Microscopically, these tumors are made up of a proliferating connective stroma and an atypical multiplication of ducts and acini, involving several lobules. The two components vary greatly in amount and provide a great variety of structure. In some adenofibromas, the epithelial component is so dominant that they might be regarded as pure adenomas.[3] The fibroblasts that form the stroma of these tumors maintain the characteristics of benign cells. Sometimes stromal changes appear, and these tumors lead to the diagnosis of cystosarcoma phyllodes, which are found in the older woman.

2.2.4. Relationship of Benign Breast Diseases to Carcinoma

Since the epithelial component of adenofibroma is presumably subject to the same biological stimuli as the breast epithelium in general, it might be expected that carcinoma might occasionally originate within an adenofibroma. In fact, very few cases have been reported, and this event is not considered as an important phenomenon.[3,11] However, the question of the eventual development of carcinoma in the breasts of patients who previously had adenofibroma remains another matter and will be discussed below.

The relationship of fibrocystic disease to mammary cancer has been extensively discussed. Prospective studies reported a 2–7 times greater frequency of cancer arising in breasts with previous evidence of fibrocystic disease.[2,4,12] Foote and Stewart[13] found that 2.5% of 1200 patients with breast cancer had a previous biopsy revealing benign breast disease, whereas only 1.1% of 120 patients with cancer elsewhere had a previous biopsy that revealed benign disease.

It is a fact that fibrocystic disease is found with high frequency in the vicinity of mammary cancer.[11] However, there is little information concerning the existence of identifiable subgroups of patients with mastopathy to which the increased risk is restricted. Humphrey and Swerdlow[14] found a correlation between duct papillomatosis with atypical features and carcinoma, but Fisher[11] found only a negligible incidence of intraductal papillomas in the vicinity of cancer in 1000 cases. Black et al.[15] showed that atypia of ductal cells in a mastopathy was a good predictor of subsequent cancer. Finally, lobular hyperplasia might also be considered as a premalignant lesion, since it appears to represent the lobular analogue of papillomatosis of larger ducts. [11] In fact, Wellings *et al.* [7] found that atypical lobules were precancerous or at least a marker for high-risk cancer tissue.

The possibility that morphological and ultrastructural studies of fibrocystic disease might provide information concerning this relationship is obvious. First, there is morphological evidence that most lesions grouped as mammary dysplasia or fibrocystic disease arose in terminal ductal lobular units or in the lobules themselves *as* the lobular and the ductal carcinoma *in situ*. [7]

Second, Fisher[11] performed a chromosome study in cells of proliferative fibrocystic disease and found karyotypic abnormalities similar to those found in examples of overt cancer. This author also found ultrastructural changes in some cases of hyperplastic fibrocystic disease analogous to those encountered in cancer, and he underlines the difficulty in the pathological distinction between atypical hyperplasia and cancer. His information represents strong evidence in support of views indicating the premalignant nature of proliferative fibrocystic disease.

3. Hormone Dependence of Benign Breast Disease

3.1. Normal Breast

Although prolactin plays an important role in the growth of mammary tumors in rodents, it does not appear to play a role in the genesis and maintenance of human breast cancer and benign breast disease. [16-19]

On the other hand, a carcinogenic role for estradiol in the breast has been suspected for a long time, particularly in animals. [17] The discovery in human breast cancers of receptors specific for estradiol and progesterone supports the thesis of hormone dependence of cancer growth. [20,21] It is known, in addition, that the presence and concentration of receptors in a mammary tumor can predict, to a certain extent, whether suppression of endogenous estrogens will have a favorable therapeutic effect. [20,21]

Such specific estradiol and progesterone receptors have not yet been demonstrated in the normal breast, although they have been found in normal uterine tissue. For this reason, among others, the hormonal dependence of breast tissue is less well explored than that of the uterus. However, proliferative and mitogenic effects of estradiol have been found in breast tissue. Estradiol is the hormone initially responsible for the differentiation and development of the ductal epithelium, increasing mitotic activity in the cylindrical cells of the internal layer of the ducts. [6,8,22] The connective tissue around the ducts, too, is very sensitive to the action of estrogen. Under estrogen stimulation, it secretes a watery mucoid sustance that has a tendency toward hyalinization.[9]

Progesterone acts, in the breast as well as in the endometrium, as both a complement and an antagonist to estradiol. Synergistically with estrogens, it acts on the distal part of the duct, favoring differentiation into acini. It therefore ensures the organization of the mammary gland for its secretory function. But progesterone is also an antiestrogen that can antagonize the action of estradiol on duct cells by changing the proliferative estrogen effects into a phase of cellular differentiation and mitotic rest.[23] In addition, progesterone induces estradiol dehydrogenase activity in human endometrium [24] and possibly in mammary glandular tissue. This leads to accelerated metabolism of estradiol to estrone, which leaves the tissue and is further metabolized into estriol. Biochemical evidence of the antiestrogenic activity of progesterone particularly its ability to decrease the concentration of estradiol receptors, has not yet been demonstrated in the breast, although it has been in the endometrium,[25] for the reason mentioned above (Table I).

In human physiology, the existence of a harmonious ovarian cyclic function ensures a perfect mammary development. In particular, the presence every month of a corpus luteum that secretes a sufficient quantity of progesterone for a normal duration of time permits a coherent organization of the galactophoric system and of the adjacent connective tissue.

Table I
Data on the Antiestrogenic Activity of Progesterone

Mode of action	Authors
Inhibition of the replenishment of cytoplasmic estradiol receptor in rat uterus	Hsueh et al. (1976)[25]
Decrease of estradiol receptor levels in human endometrium by progestins	Tseng et al. (1977)[24]
Stimulation of 17β-dehydrogenase activity in human endometrium	Tseng et al. (1977)[24]
Inhibition of epithelial-cell growth and multiplication in cultured endometrial cells of rat	Gerschenson et al. (1977)[94]

3.2. Experimental Data

In females at puberty, the mammary gland begins a growth phase that includes an increase in connective tissue, an increase in vascularity, and in some instances an increase in the deposit of adipose tissue. However, the epithelial ducts are foremost among the structures that proliferate. This proliferation is mediated through estrogens and progesterone secreted by the ovaries. Estradiol is thought to stimulate growth of the duct system, whereas lobular development depends on progesterone.[26] The basis of this conclusion is provided by many experimental observations.[27] Generally, in the species in which the cycle consists essentially of a follicular phase, the mammary gland contains primarily a ductile system. Well-developed alveoli, on the other hand, are found for the most part only in species that have a definite luteal phase. Many investigations have shown that the mammary gland of different species reacts differently to estrogen when the hormone is administered in physiological or supraphysiological doses.[8] Bässler[8] showed that large doses of estrogen administered for a long time to castrated female rats induced in the glandular tissue proliferation and dilatation of the lobules with formation of cysts and overgrowth of the epithelium. In addition, estrogen provoked an increase of circumcanalicular and intralobular connective tissue.

The time sequence of mammary morphological alteration following the administration of estradiol to female rats is: proliferation of tubular system, secretion, dilatation of ducts, formation of cysts, and fibrosis (Table II). These changes observed under the effect of supraphysiological doses of estrogen seem to be comparable with human fibrocystic disease.[8] In contrast, when estradiol is administered to castrated female rats in combination with progesterone, complete and proper development of the mammary gland is observed when the ratio between estrogen and progesterone is adequate. Cowie *et al.*[28] found in castrated goats that combination of hexoestriol and progesterone resulted in uni-

Table II
Temporal Relationship between the Effect of Estrogen and Morphogenesis of the Breast[a]

Proliferation of the tubular system	26th day
Secretion	40–60th days
Dilatation of ducts	60–90th days
Formation of cysts up to 1 cm in diameter	90–150th days
Fibrosing	150–180th days

[a]From Eisen (1942).[95] Estrogen was administered by implantation of estradiol propionate, 1–20 mg, for up to 27 months in rats.

form development and secretion when the dose of estrogen remained small (0.25 mg/day). An increase of the estrogen dose to 1 mg/day produced cysts and epithelial proliferation.

In 1941, Lyons and McGinty[29] demonstrated that the administration of estrone to immature male rabbits produced good duct growth with almost negligible alveolar formation. When animals were treated with the same dose of estrone plus increasing doses of progesterone, these authors observed that high doses of progesterone counteracted mammary-duct ectasia induced by estrogen alone and permitted, on the contrary, extensive alveolar proliferation. The antagonistic activities of estrogen and progesterone on connective tissue are also well documented.[9] Whereas the injection of estrogen into some animals induces an increase in the mucopolysaccharide content, particularly the hyaluronic acid content, in all connective tissues, progesterone appears to have an opposite effect.[9]

3.3. Ovarian Function in Women with Benign Breast Disease

Between 1972 and 1978, 550 patients with various benign breast diseases have been observed in this department. In addition to clinical, mammographic, thermographic, and cytological examinations, an endocrine study was carried out on each patient. First the basal body temperature (BBT) was recorded for 2 consecutive months; second, the endocrine function of the corpus luteum in the case of ovulating patients was evaluated.

Among the 550 patients seen for breast diseases, we paid particular attention to 309 patients who had apparent ovulatory cycles. This presumption was based on BBT measurements showing a nadir followed by a luteal plateau lasting for 8–12 days. The length of cycles studied varied between 24 and 40 days. The other 241 patients had either anovulatory cycles or cycles of more than 40 days and clear evidence of an ovulatory disorder.

The *first study* concerned 109 women between 18 and 40 years of age. They comprised 47 cases of severe incapacitating mastodynia that did not demonstrate a mass either clinically or mammographically, 28 cases of cystic mastitis authenticated by mammography followed by aspiration, and finally, 34 cases of adenofibromas demonstrated by mammography with negative aspirations. All of them were suffering from mastodynia for all or part of the cycle. All these patients presented a presumable ovulatory cycle varying in length from 24 to 40 days.

One blood sample for progesterone and estradiol assay was collected from each of the 109 patients between the first and last days of their thermal plateau. The same determinations were carried out on 50 normal women of similar age with regular 28- to 30-day cycles and a 14-day thermal plateau. In these normal women, one or two blood samples were collected between day 1 and day 13 of the thermal plateau to have 5–9 progesterone and estradiol values for each day of the luteal phase.

Plasma progesterone and estradiol were assayed by radioimmunoassay as described previously.[30] As shown in Fig. 2, wide individual variations were observed in the plasma progesterone values of normal women, particularly in the high values. However, no proges-

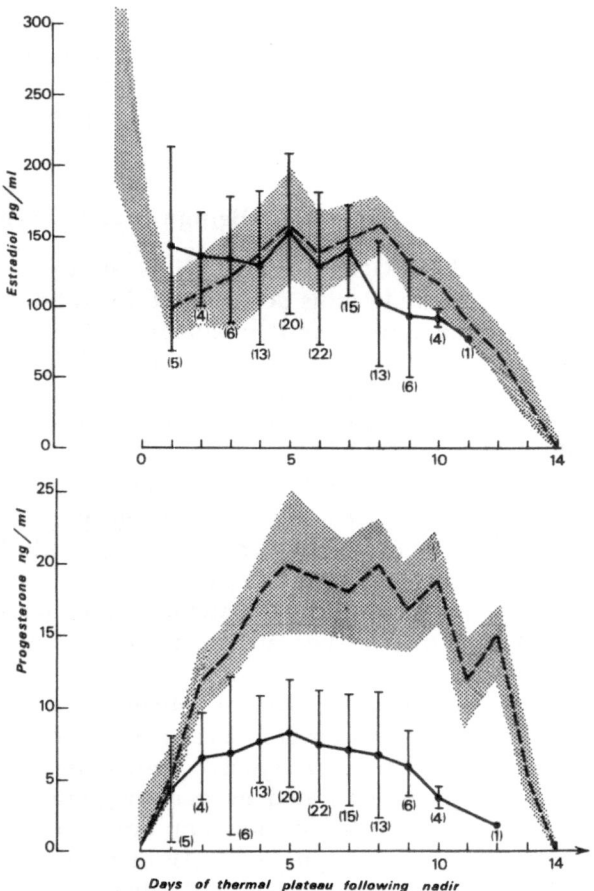

Fig. 2. Plasma estradiol and progesterone values (means ± S.E.) in 109 patients with benign breast disease studied from day 1 to day 12 of thermal plateau. The numbers in parentheses are the numbers of determinations on each day. The shaded areas indicate the means ± S.E. for plasma estradiol and progesterone values in 50 normal women studied at the same time of the menstrual cycle.

terone level lower than 10 ng/ml was observed between days 3 and 11 of the luteal phase. When daily values of plasma progesterone of patients were compared with those of normal women, it appeared that except for day 1 of the thermal plateau, all patients' levels are significantly lower ($p < 0.001$). In contrast, no significant difference was noted between daily estradiol levels of patients and those of normal women ($p > 0.5$). These results obtained from a group of patients gathered with no specification as to the type of breast lesions indicate the following: in patients with breast disease (whatever its clinical expression), plasma progesterone is generally low during the luteal phase, whereas at the same period plasma estradiol levels are within the normal range.

The *second investigation*[31] was performed on 16 patients with various benign breast diseases studied daily during the luteal phase. A blood sample was collected from each patient every day during the thermal plateau for estradiol and progesterone determinations. In these patients studied individually and on a "longitudinal basis," one can observe in 8 cases a hormonal outline very similar to that observed in the 109 patients studied "in group" (Fig. 3A), i.e., luteal levels of plasma progesterone lower than in the normal women and normal plasma estradiol levels.

In contrast, in 5 cases, plasma progesterone levels were not very different from those observed in normal women, whereas plasma estradiol levels were really elevated (more than 200 pg/ml from day 2 to

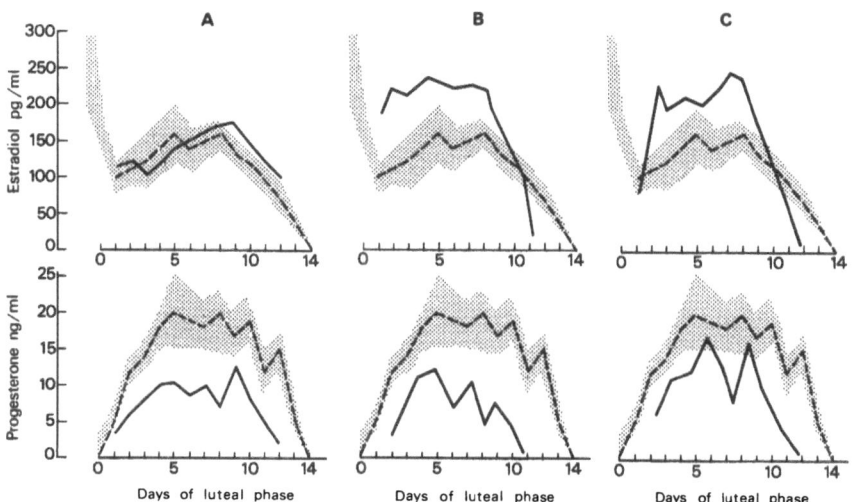

Fig. 3. Daily values of plasma progesterone and estradiol in three groups of women with benign breast disease studied during the presumed luteal phase compared with the mean ±S.E. in 50 normal women (shaded area). (A) 8 cases; (B) 3 cases; (C) 5 cases.

day 8 of the thermal plateau) (Fig. 3C). Last, in 3 cases, plasma estradiol levels were high and progesterone levels were uniformly low during the luteal phase (Fig. 3B).

In one case studied throughout a menstrual cycle of 25 days (Fig. 4), one can observe that the preovulatory peak of estradiol was 2 days late and lower than that of normal women, whereas during the luteal period estradiol was higher and progesterone lower than in the normal women.

The *third study*[19] was performed in 184 patients who were gathered into five groups according to clinical features and compared to normal women. None of them had taken any medication for at least 2 months before the study (Fig. 5).

All the patients of the five different groups were suffering from mastodynia during all or part of the cycle. Blood samples for plasma progesterone and estradiol estimation were collected from each patient at 8 A.M. three times between the first and last day of the thermal plateau, on days 5, 7, and 9.

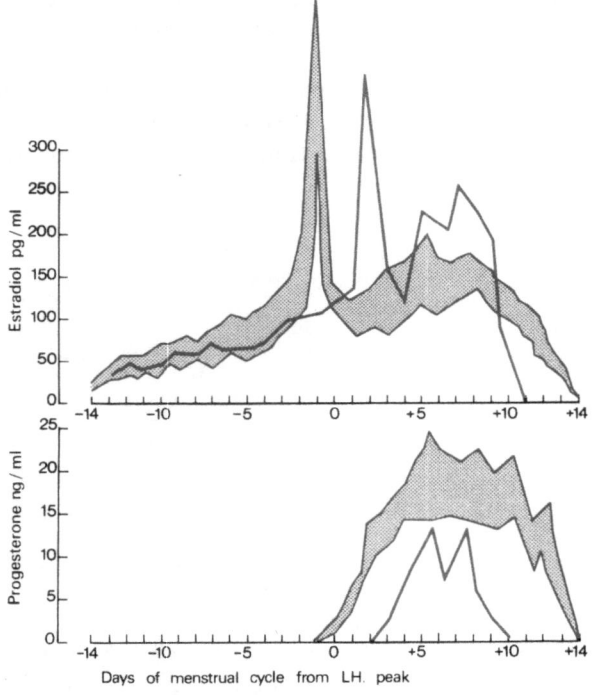

Fig. 4. Plasma levels of estradiol and progesterone studied daily throughout a 25-day cycle in a patient with mastodynia and increased nodularity of both breasts compared with the mean ±S.E. in 50 normal women (shaded area). Heavy lines denote cases.

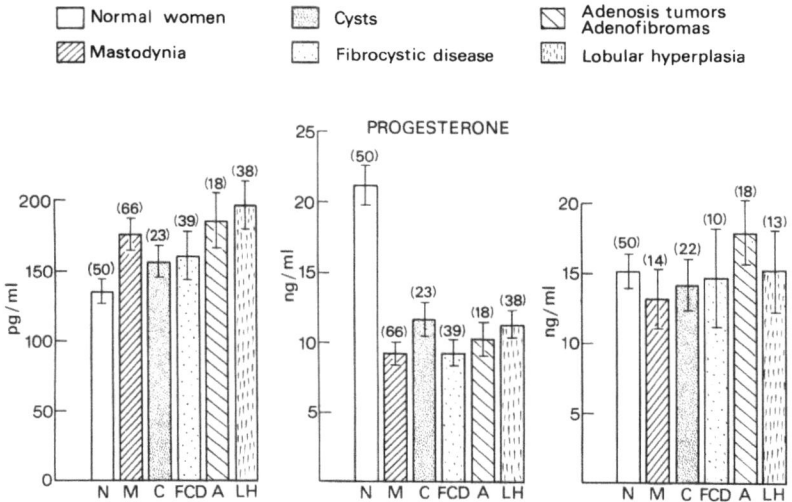

Fig. 5. Plasma levels of estradiol, progesterone, and prolactin during the luteal phase in groups of patients with mastodynia (M), isolated cysts (C), fibrocystic disease (FCD), adenofibromas (A), and increased nodularity of both breasts [lobular hyperplasia (LH)] compared to 50 normal women (N).

Plasma samples were pooled and the assay was determined from the pooled source. All the patients were also sampled once for prolactin measurement.

Plasma concentrations of progesterone, estradiol, and prolactin were calculated for each group of mastopathies and compared with those of normal women (Fig. 5).

The levels of plasma prolactin observed in the whole group of patients (15 ± 1.0 ng/ml) did not differ significantly from the levels observed in normal women (15 ± 1.2 ng/ml). In addition, no difference was noted between any group of patients and normal women.

As regards plasma progesterone, the observed values were uniformly lower than those of normal women, without any significant difference from one group of patients to another.

Plasma estradiol levels were in the normal range in patient groups I, II, and III, respectively: isolated mastodynia, cysts, and fibrocystic disease. However, they were significantly higher than in the normal women ($p < 0.01$) in groups IV and V, respectively: patients with adenofibromas and patients with increased nodularity of the breasts.

To investigate whether a correlation between plasma progesterone and estradiol levels existed during the luteal phase, the ratio of the mean plasma progesterone over the mean estradiol level observed during the luteal phase [P.E.L. = progesterone (P)/estradiol (E₂) during the luteal phase] was calculated as follows:

$$P.E.L. = \frac{P \ (pg/ml)}{E_2 \ (pg/ml)} \times 0.01$$

In the normal women, the P.E.L. ratio was 1.68 ± 0.14, while in the whole group of 184 patients this ratio was significantly lower: 0.66 ± 0.03 ($p < 0.0005$). When the individual progesterone and estradiol levels were plotted without reference to clinical features, we noted a wide distribution of the points (Fig. 6), while the representation of the individual P.E.L. values was of higher significance (Fig. 7). The P.E.L. ratio was also established for each group of breast diseases. The highest ratio (0.8 ± 0.09) was found for the patients with cystic mastitis (group II), while the lowest (0.6 ± 0.04) was observed in the patients with isolated mastodynia. These data point out the importance of evaluating the corpus luteum function of women by three plasma samples collected on

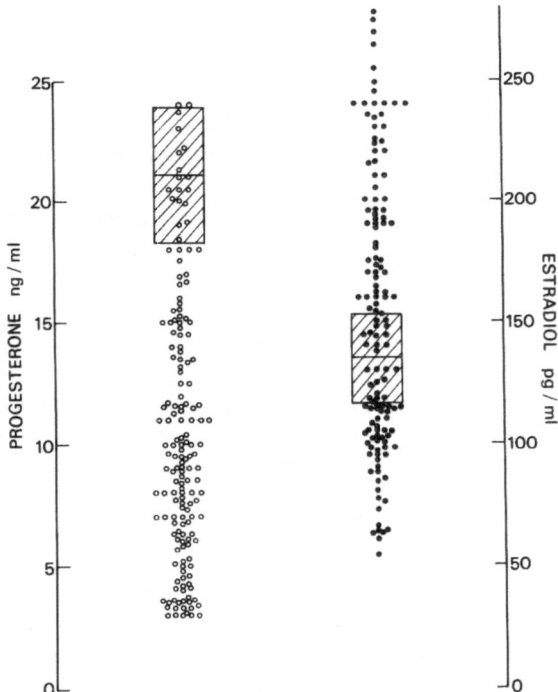

Fig. 6. Individual plasma progesterone (○) and estradiol (●) levels in 184 patients. The hatched areas indicate the means ± S.E.M. evaluated in 50 normal women.

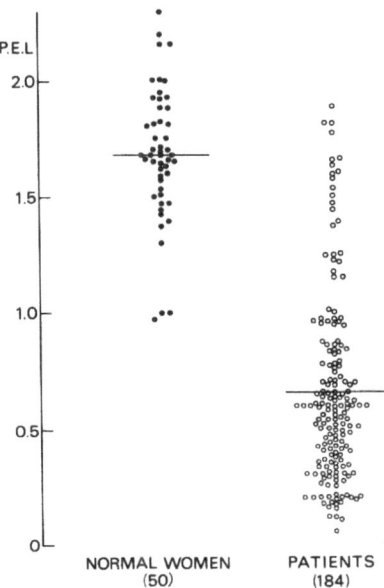

Fig. 7. Plasma progesterone level over estradiol level during the luteal phase (P.E.L.) in 184 patients (○) compared to 50 normal women (●).

days 5, 7, and 9 of the thermal plateau. This completely agrees with data obtained from the study of normal women by Abraham *et al.*[32] In addition, it appears likely that a determination of the ratio of mean plasma progesterone level over mean estradiol level in the luteal phase gives objective information about the actual steroid balance between estradiol and progesterone from the corpus luteum.

3.4. *In Vitro* Studies in Benign Breast Disease

While the presence of estradiol and progesterone receptors in breast cancer is well documented,[20,21,33,34] there is little information concerning the presence of receptors in benign breast diseases.[35-37] There are two possible explanations for the frequent absence or the small concentration of several steriod receptors in noncancerous breast tissue: first, benign breast diseases are not hormone-dependent; second, breast tissue is a very heterogenous tissue in which the receptive structures (i.e., ducts and acini) are spread into the connective tissue. The answer to these questions might be found by looking for the receptors only in the receptive cells of breast tumors obtained surgically and carefully isolated from connective tissue. The aim of our investigation was to determine whether the abnormal hormonal status observed *in vivo* by our group was correlated *in vitro* with an abnormal concentration of cytoplasmic estradiol and progesterone receptors in breast tissue.

A total of 87 women aged 15–55 years with a breast adenofibroma were studied. Plasma estradiol levels were determined on days 5, 6, and 7 of the thermal plateau and were found to be higher than that of normal women (about 300 pg/ml). Plasma progesterone values were lower than normal values, as in our previous studies.

The cellular density of the tumor was assessed by determination of the relative proportion of epithelial and stromal cells. The degrees of cellular density were distinguished. In type I, the proliferation of the acinar epithelial cells was predominant and fibrosis practically absent; in type III, the fibrosis was so predominant that the original lobular proliferation could scarcely be recognized as an adenofibroma. In type II, microscopic features were intermediate between types I and III. High-affinity binding of estradiol and progesterone was determined according to three methods: (1) sucrose gradient density; (2) a dextran-coated charcoal (DCC) assay that measures empty sites only; and (3) a method that allows the exchange of bound hormone with [^{3}H]hormone in order to determine total estradiol and progesterone receptor binding sites (E-R and P-R). [38,39]

3.4.1. Estradiol Receptors

The highest E-R levels were found in 18 adenofibromas with a very marked cellular density (41.2 ± 24.3 fmol/mg protein). In 24 adenofibromas that had an intermediate type II cellular density, the mean E-R level was 18.7 ± 11.4 fmol/mg protein, whereas in 46 adenofibromas with predominant fibrosis (type III), the mean E-R level was lower than 5 fmol/mg protein (Fig. 8).

The greatest concentrations of estradiol binding sites were observed in young patients aged from 18 to 32 years (Fig. 9) and in cases with a short length of evolution of the tumor at the time of surgery (15 days to 5 months). In contrast, patients with a low concentration of estradiol binding sites (L-ER) were older (32–55 years) and the length of evolution of their tumors was more than 9 months (Fig. 10). In the medium group (M-ER), the age and the length of evolution were intermediate. In other words, the greatest concentration of estradiol binding sites was observed in tumors with high epithelial cellularity and that had developed recently. This condition was particularly observed in young women. A similar observation was made by Rosen *et al.*[37] in a shorter series of 23 adenofibromas.

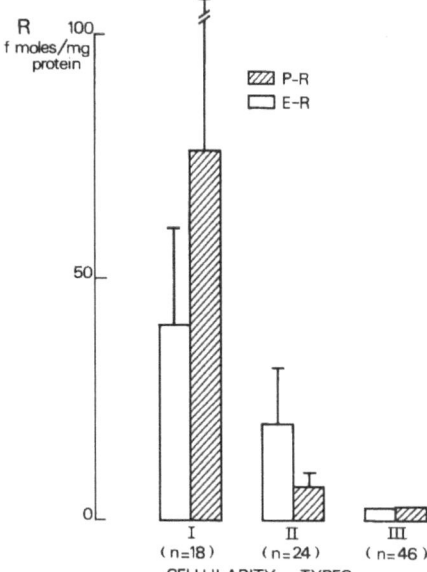

Fig. 8. Cytosol estradiol binding sites (E–R) and progesterone binding sites (P-R) levels in three groups of adenofibromas according to their epithelial cell density: high in group I (n = 18), medium in group II (n = 24), and low in group III (n = 46).

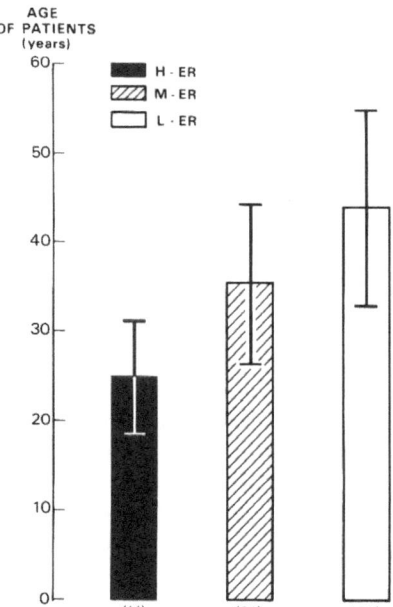

Fig. 9. Age distribution of patients in the three groups of adenofibromas: H–ER [estradiol binding sites (ER) > 20 fmol/mg protein], M–ER (ER > 7 to < 20 fmol/mg protein), and L–ER (ER < 7 fmol/mg protein).

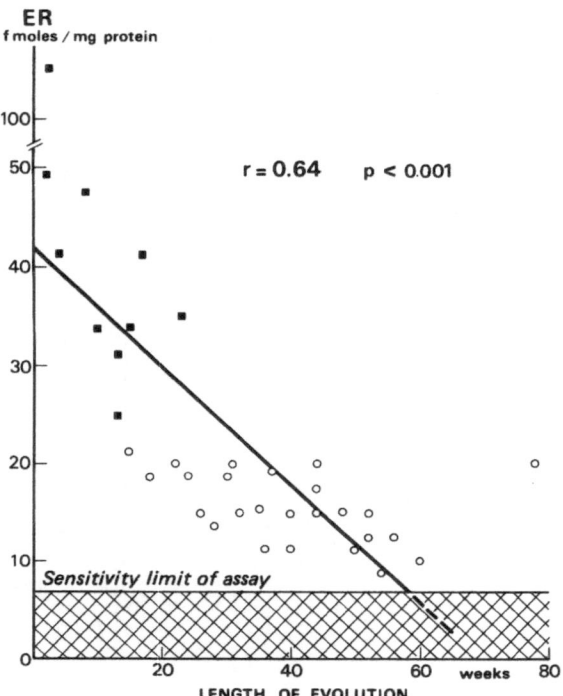

Fig. 10. Linear correlation ($p < 0.001$) between the estradiol cytosol binding sites (ER) calculated from Scatchard plots after DCC-exchange assays (ER $= y$) and the length of the
adenofibroma evolution between discovery and surgery (x) in the 11 patients of the H–ER
group (■) and the 24 patients of the M–ER group (○). The limit of sensitivity of the assay
is ER $= 7$ fmol/mg cytosolic protein.

3.4.2. *Progesterone Receptors*

As regards progesterone receptors, P-R levels were constantly elevated in type I adenofibromas (76.9 ± 54 fmol/mg protein) (see Fig. 8).
They were low in the two other groups of adenofibromas: 6.0 ± 3.7 and
less than 5 fmol/mg protein in groups II and III, respectively.

It is interesting that breast tissue was obtained at midfollicular
phase. At this period of the cycle, estradiol production is elevated and
there is no substantial secretion of progesterone by the ovary. These two
conditions are necessary to allow a high synthesis of P-R and no translo-
cation to the nucleus. [21]

As shown in Fig. 11, there is no parallelism between P-R and E-R
levels. However, if P-R levels are plotted as a function of E-R levels,

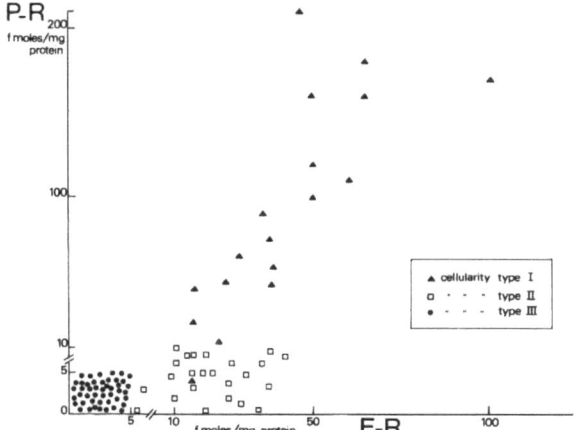

Fig. 11. Correlation between estradiol and progesterone cytosol binding sites (ER and PR) in the three groups of adenofibromas: (▲) type I, with high epithelial cellular density; (□) type II, with medium epithelial cellular density; (●) type III, with low epithelial cellular density.

three different areas can be distinguished that correspond closely to the three cellular types of tumor: (1) adenofibromas with elevated levels of both E-R and P-R correspond to type I cellularity; (2) adenofibromas with medium E-R levels and low P-R levels correspond to cellularity type II; and (3) adenofibromas with both E-R and P-R levels under 5 fmol/mg protein correspond to type III cellularity ($p < 0.1$).

3.4.3. Interpretation of Results

The presence of estradiol and progesterone receptors in the adenofibromas with great cellular density gives additional support to the hypothesis that benign breast diseases are estrogen-dependent. Previously, Cortes-Gallegos et al.[40] found a higher concentration of estradiol in breast tissue from patients with benign mastopathy than in normal breast tissue (Table III).

In addition, progesterone receptors were observed only in the group of adenofibromas with high epithelial cellularity and very little fibrosis. Most of these tumors had been discovered early in young women, and surgery was performed shortly after diagnosis. The fact that in these recent tumors both estradiol and progesterone receptors were present indicates that cell differentiation remains normal insofar as there is no stromal reaction characterized by an intralobular fibrosis of the mantle tissue.[8]

Table III
Estradiol Content of Different Human
Breast Tissues[a]

Mammary gland tissue	Estradiol (pg/g tissue) (mean)
Normal	1365
Gynecomastia	1705
Cystic breast disease	3659

[a]From Cortes-Gallegos *et al.*[40] (1975)

The observation in adenofibromas of a persistent estrogen dependence without the presence of progesterone receptors is interesting to consider, since P-R is an index of estrogen sensitivity of target cells and reflects their differentiated and functional state. It appears that in group II (E-R+, P-R −), cell "dedifferentiation" has occurred. This "dedifferentiation" would result not only in the loss of P-R as a functional marker, but also in a relative insensitivity of the adenofibroma cell to the physiological regulation of endogenous progesterone. However, from all these results, it may be postulated that insofar as all benign breast diseases have the same hormonal characteristics as those observed in adenofibromas, the treatment of these lesions by progesterone or progestins or both may be effective before the appearance of fibrosis—in other words, in recent lesions that are still hormone-dependent, this hormone dependence being attested *in vitro* by the presence of at least estradiol receptors.

3.5. Hormonal Treatment of Benign Breast Disease

3.5.1. Introduction

A total of 380 patients with benign breast disease and with a hormonal profile characteristic of an inadequate luteal phase or anovulatory cycles have been treated in our department by progesterone and progestins. This treatment was prescribed to correct their defect in the ovarian secretion of progesterone. This therapeutic experience began 5 years ago and is at present being followed up.[41]

The 380 patients on whom a progestogen treatment was undertaken had various mammary symptoms as regards their type and their importance. Some had only one symptom; most had an association of symptoms.

To have more precise information on the effects of the treatment, it seemed to us more objective to estimate the results obtained in relation to a given mammary symptom than to calculate the results obtained on a group of symptoms. Under these conditions, this study concerned 620 symptom manifestations observed in 380 patients. The following symptoms were manifested:

- 249 cases of mastodynia defined as: bilateral incapacitating breast pain either premenstrual or continuous but with postmenstrual improvement.
- 115 cases in which clinical examination showed increased nodularity of both breasts that did not disappear after menstruation. In these cases, mammography denotes dense breasts with a predominant ductal pattern. There were neither cysts nor adenomas, but large plates of sclerosis.
- 63 cases of fibrocystic disease of both breasts diagnosed by mammography and needle aspiration.
- 122 cases of isolated cysts authenticated by mammography followed by aspiration.
- 71 cases of adenofibromas demonstrated by mammography with negative needle aspiration.

3.5.2. Treatment Scheme

All the patients were treated with sequential administration of progestins given orally and progesterone topically applied to both breasts.

At the beginning of this therapeutical experience, some of the patients were treated with either oral progestins or topical progesterone. Since we observed that the association was significantly more efficient than each treatment alone,[42] we went on with the study using the combined progesterone–progestin treatment.

- The progestin was Lynestrenol, 10 mg/day, from day 10 to day 25 of the menstrual cycle. The duration of this treatment varied from 9 months to 4 years.
- The percutaneous application of progesterone consisted of an alcohol water gel in which the steroid was dissolved. Progesterone, 50 mg, was applied to the breast daily.

It has been previously demonstrated that radioactive progesterone topically applied can be absorbed through the skin. Indeed, labeled metabolites (pregnanediol and allopregnanediol) were recovered in the 48-hr urine after percutaneous administration of the precursor.[43] We had also calculated[43] that percutaneous absorption of the steroid was low, only 10%. Therefore, the daily administration of 50 mg progesterone might result in a local concentration of 5 mg active progesterone.

Recent *in vitro* studies from this laboratory confirm the presence of significantly higher levels of progesterone in breasts than in peripheral blood after percutaneous administration of this steriod (unpublished data). This has also been recently demonstrated by de Boever *et al.*,[44] who found local concentrations of progesterone 3 times higher in breast tissue of patients treated with percutaneous progesterone than in controls.

Moreover, the high fat solubility of progesterone is responsible for a prolonged local retention of the steroid. In addition, because of an extensive *in situ* metabolism of progesterone in the breast,[43,45] there was no systemic effect of the steroid, in particular no significant modification in endometrial histology and no breakthrough bleeding.

De Boever *et al.*[44] also found no increase in plasma level of progesterone after percutaneous application of the steroid despite its high local concentrations in the mammary gland.

For all these reasons, percutaneous progesterone was administered every day including during the menstrual period.

Indeed, the fact that progesterone is continuously present inside the breast might permit a permanent antiestrogenic effect, which competes with the eventual presence of a high local estradiol concentration.[40] In addition, the administration of 10 mg Lynestrenol a day results in a substantial decrease in gonadotropin secretion and in plasma concentration of estradiol (Figs. 12 and 13). This result is of importance because

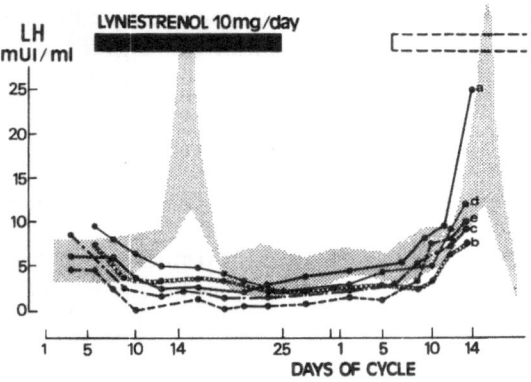

Fig. 12. Daily plasma luteinizing hormone (LH) levels of five normal women during the administration of 10 mg Lynestrenol from day 5 to day 25 of the menstrual cycle. The shaded area represents the untreated cycle in 50 normal women.

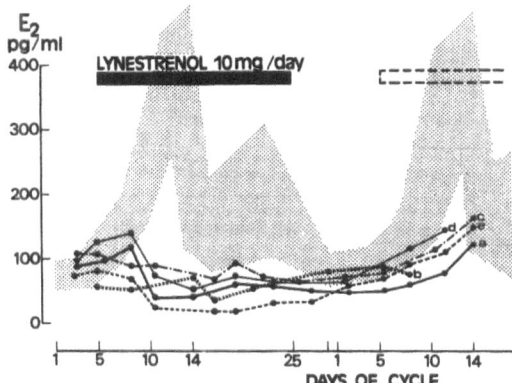

Fig. 13. Daily plasma estradiol (E2) levels of five normal women during the administration of 10 mg Lynestrenol from day 5 to day 25 of the menstrual cycle. The shaded area represents the untreated cycle in 50 normal women.

Lynestrenol was also used in young women for its contraceptive effect. [46.47]

3.5.3. Results

Results obtained by combined progesterone–Lynestrenol treatment on 620 symptom manifestations relevant to diverse mastopathies are given in Table IV. The therapeutic results of hormonal treatment of benign breast disease were expressed as follows:

The beneficial effects consisted in a complete disappearance of breast pain and tenderness, in particular during the premenstrual period. Mammary glands became supple and nodularities disappeared.

On mammography, the results obtained were less clear, and there was always a disparity between clinical and radiological results. Indeed, it is difficult to obtain comparable films at two consecutive examinations. In addition, edema is not easily visualized on mammography, whereas indelible intralobular sclerosis—thicker than glandular tissue—masks the modification of glandular tissue, due to hormonal treatment. In contrast, there was a very clear improvement in vascular pictures after treatment judged by thermography[46] (Figs. 14 and 15).

The total improvement of breast pain and tenderness was observed from the very beginning of the treatment in 96% of the 249 cases of mastodynia.

The 4% failure was observed when this symptom was associated with fibrocystic disease or cysts. In fact, of the patients with fibrocystic disease, only 10% were improved with the treatment. In these cases, microcysts disappeared and did not develop again during the course of the treatment. The cysts treated first by needle aspiration did not reappear during the hormonal treatment in 50% of the cases. The adenofi-

Table IV
Results Obtained after Treatment of 380 Patients with 620 Mammary Symptom Manifestations[a]

Results	Isolated mastodynia (234 cases)	Increased nodularity (70 cases)	Isolated cysts (88 cases)	Chronic fibro-cystic disease (56 cases)	Adenofibromas (52 cases)
Good results	96%	85%	50%	10%	50%
Failures	4%	15%	50%	90%	50%

[a] The treatment was 50 mg percutaneous progesterone applied daily to the breast plus sequential administration of 10 mg Lynestrenol 15 days/cycle.

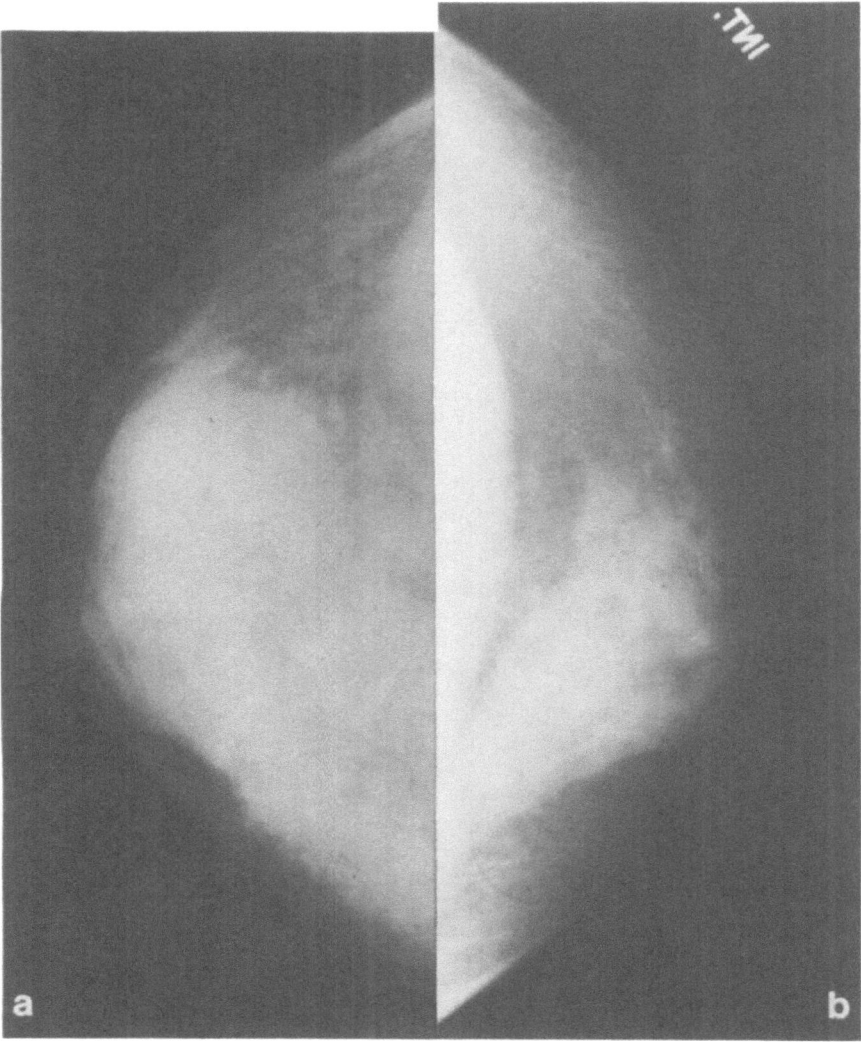

Fig. 14. Caudal projection of the left breast of a 32-year-old woman suffering from mastodynia and increased nodularity of the breasts. (a) Dense radiographic appearance before treatment; (b) disappearance of most of the cloudy areas after 3 months' treatment with percutaneous progesterone.

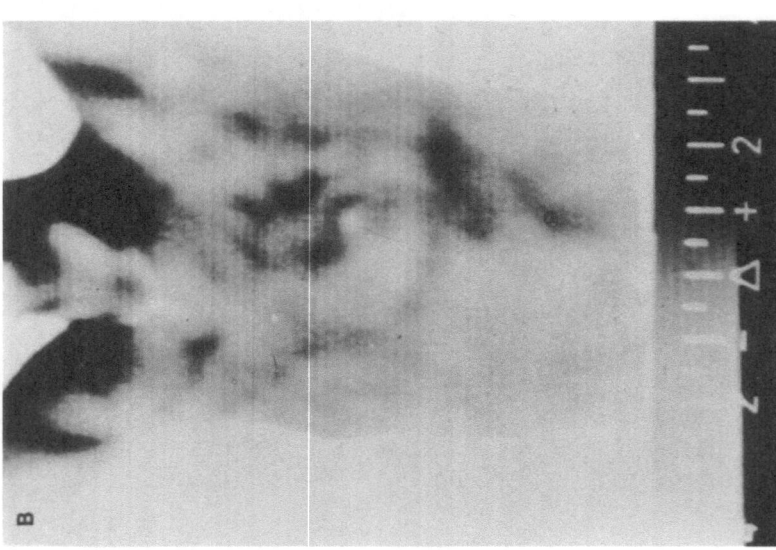

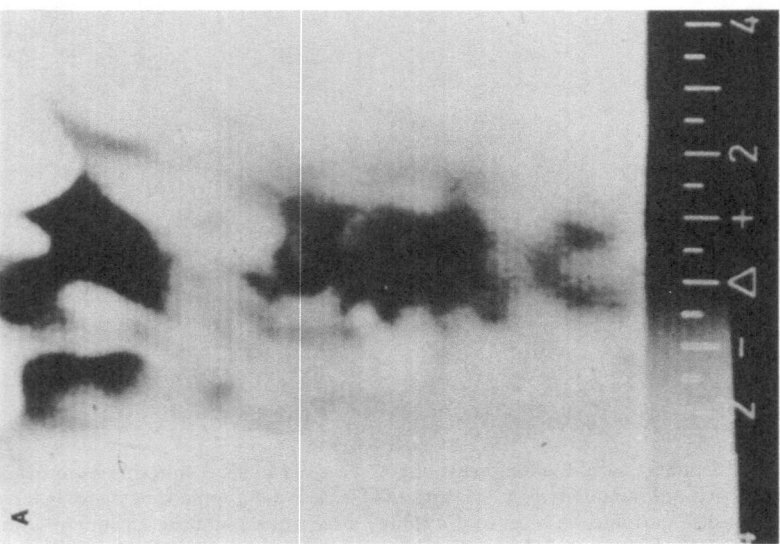

Fig. 15. (A) Telethermography in a 23-year-old woman suffering from increased nodularity of the upper outer section of the left breast. The vascular pattern is enlarged with hyperthermia of most of the left breast. (B) After 3 months' treatment with percutaneous progesterone plus Lynestrenol, most of the vascular abnormalities are corrected.

bromas were largely reduced or disappeared in 50% of the cases. A high rate of improvement (85%) was observed in the cases of increased nodularity of the breasts. In these cases, the lesions completely disappeared, and in the remaining 15%, no improvement was observed. In these last cases, the lesions had been present for many years and were far larger than in the cases where the treatment was effective.

It appears clear that the higher percentage of beneficial results was obtained with this treatment on symptoms ascribable to recent lesions, in particular in the case of isolated mastodynia, in which treatment was also invariably effective. The results of this treatment were also remarkable in the case where increased nodularity of the breasts had recently appeared, and in which sclerosis was either absent or only slight.

Some positive results were also obtained in "young" adenofibromas. This confirms our *in vitro* data showing that estradiol and progesterone receptors were found only in adenofibromas with considerable cellularity and no fibrosis.[38,39] It was possible to establish a correlation between the presence of progesterone receptors in "young" adenofibromas and the response to hormonal treatment.

In contrast, "old" adenofibromas with marked fibrosis and poor cellularity did not respond to the treatment with progestrone and progestins. This is also the case in chronic fibrocystic disease in which sclerosis is the main histological component. The presence of estradiol or progesterone receptors was not assayed in this type of disease. However, indirectly, the negative results obtained by the progestational treatment might indicate that in this sort of chronic disease, hormone dependence had ceased for a long time previously.

3.5.4. Interpretation of Results

These results lead to the following considerations:

Hormonal treatment of benign breast diseases is effective if it is begun very soon in the course of the disease, particularly in the case where unopposed estrogen action is responsible only for edema and reversible glandular hyperplasia. For these reasons, we estimate that mastodynia is not a physiological event but is probably the first symptom of a hyperestrogenic milieu inside the breast.[22]

Moreover, benign breast disease not only must be treated at the beginning of its history but also should be treated for a long time, in particular in the case where the disease is associated with another risk factor for breast cancer.

3.5.5. Other Hormonal Treatment of Benign Breast Disease

Other authors tried successfully to treat benign breast diseases with Danazol.[48-50] In fact, this molecule is a synthetic analogue of ethinyl testosterone and exerts its therapeutic effects mainly through its inhibitory action on gonadotropin secretion.[51] Thus, it has been proposed for the treatment of endometriosis[52] and also for contraception.[53] It has also been recently suggested that Danazol exerts a direct action on the ovary leading to an inhibition of steroidogenesis.[54]

Since the aim of this treatment is to obtain a high antiestrogenic activity in the mammary gland, it may be compared to the progestin treatment action. The clinical results[48] seem comparable with the two treatments.

However, the side effects of Danazol treatment are considerable because of its anabolic and androgenic properties.[53] At least in our experience, these effects have been worse than those observed in patients treated with progestins.[46]

At the moment, in this department, we are conducting a survey of more than 1000 patients. The aim of this survey is to discover whether patients treated over a period of 10 years would have a lower risk of breast cancer than the untreated ones.

3.6. Pathophysiological Interpretation of the Hormonal Abnormalities Observed in Women with Benign Breast Disease

3.6.1. Inadequate Corpus Luteum Function

The existence of an inadequate corpus luteum was first observed in oligomenorrheic women with reduced fertility.[55] This inadequate corpus luteum is characterized by an abnormally low progesterone secretion contrasting with normal estradiol values and is a result of a disorder in gonadotropin secretion. The concentration of follicle-stimulating hormone (FSH) is below normal during the follicular phase, while the preovulatory and ovulatory secretion of luteinizing hormone (LH) is normal.

At the same time, Backström and Cartensen[56] and Backström *et al.*[57] observed that women with premenstrual tension had elevated concentrations of plasma estradiol and low plasma progesterone levels during the luteal phase.

There is only limited information about the true action of estradiol and progesterone in breast physiology and pathology in human beings. This may be explained as follows: It is very difficult to obtain steroid receptors in normal breast tissue and even in tissue obtained from benign breast disease.

There are only a few data on the luteal function of women with benign breast diseases. It is only recently that studies have emphasized the importance of plasma progesterone determination to estimate the corpus luteum function,[32,58,59] since it did not seem possible to rely precisely on the BBT curve and on the level of urinary pregnanediol.[31] Now there are many studies in which attempts have been made to evaluate the plasma levels of progesterone that are consistent with a normal luteal function. One can estimate that 4 days after the thermal nadir, plasma values of progesterone equal to or greater than 10 ng/ml reflect a good functional corpus luteum.[32] In contrast, great variations in plasma estradiol values are observed in a normal menstrual cycle, but usually they are between 100 and 160 pg/ml during the luteal phase. Considering these data, it appears likely that women with benign breast disease have an inadequate corpus luteum function. This progestational insufficiency in women with apparently normal cycles is important, since other women with the same mammary symptoms (45% in our series) have a monophasic BBT curve and an endometrial histology inconsistent with ovulatory cycles.[60] These women may have an absolute progestational insufficiency.

The frequency with which an inadequate corpus luteum is observed in women with benign mastopathy should warn the clinician that in judging the functional quality of the corpus luteum, he cannot be satisfied with a mere appreciation of a biphasic BBT curve. Only the ratio of plasma progesterone over plasma estradiol levels in a presumed luteal phase is able to give objective information on luteal function. It is interesting that patients with recent lesions characterized histologically by marked cellularity with little fibrosis have an increase in both plasma estradiol and receptors of estradiol and progesterone in breast tissue. However, in old lesions, there are neither elevated plasma estradiol concentrations nor detectable steroid receptors in the tissue. These data may account for the remarkable effect of the treatment with progesterone and progestins in recent benign breast lesions where cellular hyperplasia is predominant and fibrosis still absent such as isolated mastodynia, recent adenofibromas, and increased nodularity of both breasts. In fact, this treatment needs the presence of progesterone receptors to be effective; indeed, in old lesions with much fibrosis, there are no steroid receptors or only a small concentration of estradiol receptors.

The persistent estrogenic stimulation of breast tissue without the moderating and perhaps protective effects of progesterone noted in patients with benign breast diseases suggests the possibility that an estradiol vs. progesterone imbalance may play a role in the development of female genital-tract dystrophies. This assumption concerning the pathogenesis of endometrial hyperplasia and adenocarcinoma is well documented. [61] Our observations support the hypothesis that a similar hormonal stimulus may provide a propitious setting in the mammary gland for the development of benign lesions. This hypothesis is largely reinforced by our therapeutic data that indicate the usefulness of treating recent breast lesions. In contrast, the observation of normal plasma prolactin levels in patients studied by our group does not allow any conclusion as to a possible relationship between prolactin and benign breast diseases.

3.6.2. Concept of "Dysovulation"

The role of the central nervous system in provoking abnormalities of corpus luteum function observed in women with breast diseases is very likely. Indeed, inadequate corpus luteum and anovulatory cycles are essentially related to an abnormality in gonadotropin secretion.[62] Anovulatory or "dysovulatory" cycles may occur in women at any time during their reproductive life, but they are most common immediately after menarche and before menopause, both periods being characterized by a particularly high incidence of benign breast diseases[22,60] (Table V).

But ovulation can also be disturbed at any time during the reproductive life. Its cyclic hypothalamic regulation is complex, and in some women and some families it is extremely sensitive to psychological and sensorial stimuli. Emotions, aggressions, some episodes of sentimental, familial, or professional life (of which the dramatic character is quite unequally perceived) can also interfere with the ovulatory regulation.[63,64] In the words of Matsumoto *et al.*[63] : " ... The existence of

Table V
Hypothesis Concerning the Concept of Dysovulation[a]

Pathophysiology
· Inappropriate gonadotropin secretion due to a central catecholamine dysfunction[78]
Etiology
· Physiological[96]
  Postmenarche
  Perimenopause
· Pathological
  Environmental conditions[63]
  Psychological disturbances
  Individual predisposing factors[64]
Pathological consequences
· Hormonal
  Decreased production of progesterone during the luteal phase with normal or increased estradiol secretion: unopposed estrogen effect[55,97]
· Cellular
  Increased cellular multiplication[94]
· Clinical
  Premenstrual tension[57]
  Menstrual disorders[98]
  Hypofertility[55]
  Benign breast diseases[19,60,78,97]

[a]From Mauvais-Jarvis *et al.* (1979).[78]

environmental amenorrhea, such as war amenorrhea, emotional amenorrhea, detention amenorrhea and psychogenic amenorrhea is a well established theory. However, it appears that the same environmental changes in life or psychic trauma can also induce anovulatory cycles and ovulatory oligomenorrhea (retarded ovulation)!..." (p. 35). In our series of patients with benign breast diseases, such environmental factors have been very frequently noted.[31]

In addition, it was observed in practically 50% of our patients that many disorders of ovulation are clinically latent because the length of the menstrual cycle remains normal, and very often one does not attach enough importance to certain premenstrual manifestations that may be related to luteal insufficiency. Among these, premenstrual tension with anxiety[56] and breast tenderness and mastodynia[22] are particularly representative of an unopposed estrogen effect.

3.6.3. Role of Androgens

Grattarola[65] has shown that premenopausal breast cancer patients have a significantly higher frequency of anovulatory cycles than controls of similar age. In addition, he found that the excretion of testosterone was significantly increased in 10 breast cancer patients whose endometrial pattern was shown to be atypical.[66] The removed ovaries were found to have multiple cysts and hyperplasia of the ovarian interstitial tissue. Recently, Grattarola[67] found that 18 of 26 patients (64%) with fibrocystic disease of the breast showed an increased level of urinary testosterone and androstanediol (a target-organ metabolite of testosterone).[68] This observation indicated to Grattarola[69] that an abnormal androgenicity could create the condition that induces fibrocystic disease—a premalignant condition in the breast. In fact, increased androstanediol and testosterone excretion is always observed in women with polycystic ovaries,[70] and the stromal hyperplasia of the ovaries coincides with the absence, in this disease, of the ovulatory peak of LH and the lack of corpus luteum.[71] In other words, the exaggerated excretion of testosterone or androstanediol observed in patients with benign breast disease may be interpreted as the result of a disorder of the ovulatory function in premenopausal women.

4. Relationship between Benign Breast Disease and Breast Cancer

We mentioned above the predisposing role of benign breast disease in cancer. The exact evaluation remains extremely imprecise. The only useful studies concern cystic disease, which increases the risk of cancer approximately 4-fold.[2] It is very interesting, in our opinion, that a recent study from the Mayo Clinic[4] showed that a majority of cancers observed in patients with a previous history of cystic disease became clinically apparent 5–10 years after the benign disease was diagnosed. This observation was made in women 40–49 years old when their cancer was diagnosed. It confirms the notion of a long time interval between the appearance of benign dystrophy and cancer, which takes into account the likely tumor doubling time. With regard to the mechanism of the association between cancer and cystic mastitis, MacMahon *et al.*[72] give two explanations: ". . . 1) The cystic disease itself is a premalignant condition that either predisposes to neoplastic change or is an early manifestation of malignant change or 2) benign and malignant breast diseases have etiologic factors in common—perhaps a particular hormone pattern."

Recently, Bulbrook *et al.*[73] have reported the level of plasma estradiol and progesterone in women with varying degrees of risk of breast cancer. In premenopausal women, these authors noted that increased risk of breast cancer correlated with subnormal plasma progesterone values in the luteal phase of the menstrual cycle. Plasma estradiol values do not vary with risk. Another approach to the problem consists in the examination of the hormonal status of women with breast cancer. Breast cancer as well as endometrial cancer is considered to be a hormone-dependent malignancy. In some women, changes in the hormonal environment of the neoplasia have succeeded in temporarily slowing down or arresting the cancerous growth.

The risk of breast cancer increases with age. Incidence rises between the ages of 25 and 45 and levels off between 45 and 55. Thereafter, the curve of incidence resumes its upward course. Accordingly, peaks of breast cancer incidence between ages 45 and 49 and approximately 65 and 70 have been suggested.[74] Thus, the first peak of incidence of breast cancer has been related to an ovarian estrogen disturbance, whereas the increase in breast cancer incidence after age 60 is thought to be possibly due to a postmenopausal stimulus. This stimulus is either of adrenocortical origin,[74] in particular an increase in the conversion of androstenedione to estrone in extraglandular tissue,[75] or due to the intake of exogenous estrogen by postmenopausal women.[76] The risk factors for breast cancer are well known, but they are generally interpreted in different ways. Sherman and Korenman,[77] on one hand, and our group,[78] on the other, have advanced the suggestion that the main known risk factors for breast cancer may be interpreted in the same way. Both interpretations are based on the postulation that in terms of epidemiology, "unopposed estrogen effect" is carcinogenic and that adequate progesterone secretion by corpus luteum has a protecting ef-

Table VI
Factors Associated with Luteal Function That Influence Breast Cancer Risk

Factors that increase the risk of breast cancer	Factors that decrease the risk of breast cancer
Family history of breast cancer	Short fertile life (low number of menstrual cycles)
Benign breast disease	Early menopause
Early onset of menarche	Early age at first term pregnancy
Late menopause	Multiparity
Nulliparity, unmarried (?)	Bilateral ovariectomy in early fertile life
Failure of ovulation (lack of progesterone)	Low socioeconomic status
Prolonged estrogen treatment	Life in rural areas
Low urinary estriol ratio	
High socioeconomic status	
Life in urban areas	

fect against breast cancer development. Thus, by comparing the particular environment of benign breast diseases to factors considered to confer high risk for malignancy of the breast, we concluded[78] that the following factors might be interpreted as reflecting an abnormal regulation of the female reproductive cycle[78] (Table VI): (1) early menarche and late menopause; (2) nulliparity and late age at first pregnancy; (3) familial risk factors; (4) ethnic risk factors; (5) urinary estrogen abnormalities; and (6) urinary androgen-excretion abnormalities.

5. Role of Exogenous Estrogens in the Incidence of Benign Breast Disease

5.1. Oral Contraceptives

1. The *incidence of breast tumors in women who have been using oral contraceptives* is very difficult to interpret. Initial studies[79-83] failed to demonstrate an increased evidence of breast cancer in women using contraceptive steroids. In addition, very incomplete information suggests that oral contraceptive agents may exert a protective effect on the development of benign breast neoplasm.[84] Epidemiological studies, indeed, showed a lower frequency of fibrocystic disease among long-term users of oral contraceptives than among women who have never used them.[84] However, in a case control study of 452 breast cancer patients less than 50 years old, Paffenbarger *et al.*[85] observed that the relative risk of breast cancer from regular use of the pill for 2–4 years was

increased 7-fold among those women with established benign breast disease (Table VII). From their results, Paffenbarger *et al.*[85] concluded that the pill ". . . as new and different ingested material could be implicated as either inducing or promoting breast cancer in women presenting benign breast lesions . . . ." A recent prospective study from Lees *et al.*[86] leads to the same conclusion. For these authors, the use of oral contraceptives for more than 5 years by women with a prior breast biopsy for benign breast disease increases the risk of breast cancer 9-fold. Lees *et al.*[86] concluded that their results sustain the hypothesis that long-term use of oral contraceptives promotes the development of cancer in women with a history of benign breast disease. Similarly, in a more recent epidemiological study, Brinton *et al.*[87] reported that an excessive risk of breast cancer was observed in long-term users of oral contraceptives with a previous biopsy for benign breast disease. For this group, oral contraceptives also seemed to enhance the effects of other risk indicators such as family history of breast cancer and late first childbirth.

2. *A paradox concerning the relationship among oral contraceptives, breast cancer, and benign breast disease* is thus evident. Oral contraceptives appear to protect against benign breast disease,[81-84] which may itself be a risk factor for breast cancer. On the other hand, oral contraceptives evidently increase the risk of mammary carcinoma in women with a clinical history of benign breast disease. MacMahon *et al.*[72] suggest that these findings may be reconciled by a concept of two types of benign breast disease, based on the results of Black *et al.*[15] Black *et al.*[15] found that women with ductal atypia in a benign breast lesion had a higher risk of subsequent mammary carcinoma than did women with no evidence of atypical changes.

The ductal atypia in benign breast lesions may represent a premalignant condition, perhaps subject to stimulation by oral contraceptives, while the absence of ductal atypia may be characteristic of nonpremalignant forms of benign breast disease, the formation or development of which might perhaps be inhibited by oral contraceptives. Similarly, LiVolsi *et al.*[88] found, from a histopathological evaluation of 205 premenopausal women, that the assumption by which oral contraceptives protect patients with fibrocystic disease against cancer may be applied only to fibrocystic disease in which epithelial atypia is minimal or absent and not to the more developed forms of this condition. If oral contraceptives do actually suppress the development of disease with minimal or absent ductal atypia, the hormonal mechanisms remain to be determined. Among these, one can advance the theory that the utilization of an oral contraceptive perfectly fitted to an individual "hormonal milieu" may protect against the development of benign breast disease. This is

Table VII
Relative Risk of Breast Cancer Related to Use of Oral Contraceptives in Women with Prior Benign Breast Disease

Authors	Relative risk[a] according to duration of oral contraceptive use (yr)	
	<5	>5
Paffenbarger et al. (1977)[85]	1.2	11.2
Lees et al. (1978)[86]	5.0	9.0
Brinton et al. (1979)[87]	5.0	16.0

[a]Relative risk = 1.0 for women who have never used oral contraceptives.

particularly true in the case of women with inadequate luteal function. In these patients, indeed, the oral contraceptives may suppress endogenous hormone production, for instance, an excessive secretion of estradiol by ovaries. It has recently been reported[89] that the appearance of benign breast disease in women taking a combined oral contraceptive is negatively associated with the dose of the progestagen component (Table VIII).

Generally, oral contraceptive agents that contain a high concentration of progestin give a low proportion of breast engorgement and mastodynia. In fact, the choice of an adequate contraceptive is difficult. Progestins, indeed, have various biological effects; they are not only progestational but also estrogenic, antiestrogenic, and androgenic, and these different activities vary from one progestin to another. In addition,

Table VIII
Effect of Progestin Content in Oral Contraceptives on the Development of Benign Breast Disease[a]

Benign breast disease	Ethinyl estradiol, 50 μg/per day + norethisterone acetate		
	1 mg	3 mg	4 mg
Number	78	59	9
Percentage per 1000 women/ year	7.18	4.18	3.57

[a]From Royal College of General Practitioners (1977).[89]

pills differ in type and dosage of progestin and estrogen. Thus, knowledge of such potential additive or antagonist effects is important in choosing a type of oral contraceptive to adapt well to a given clinical situation.[90] These thoughts on the effective clinical potency of oral contraceptives suggest that epidemiological studies published at present cannot give valuable information on the cancer risk related to the use of oral contraceptives. Current statistics, indeed, are based on retrospective studies of insufficient length in which a variety of contraceptive agents, quite different from one another, are used. From a practical point of view, it seems that contraception based on a combination of estrogen plus progestin is contraindicated in women with benign breast disease, even only limited to a mastodynia. In these patients, progestins given 15 days a month are efficient contraceptives.[47] In our opinion, this method of contraception must also be proposed to women with a high risk of breast cancer (even in the absence of benign breast disease) and systematically to women over 40 years of age.

5.2. Estrogen Treatment of Menopausal Women

1. *A possible relationship between estrogenic hormones and carcinoma of the endometrium and breast in human beings has been suspected for many years.*[91] As for contraceptive agents, results of retrospective studies on the occurrence of breast cancer in postmenopausal women using exogenous estrogens are very conflicting. [76,92,93]

The most interesting study is that of Hoover *et al.*[76] on 1891 women who for 12 years were taking conjugated estrogen for the treatment of menopausal symptoms. The relative risk of breast cancer increased with duration of follow-up estrogen treatment, progressing to 2.0 after 15 years. The highest risk occurred in women using higher doses of estrogen and in those taking the medication on some other than a daily basis. In addition, after 10 years of follow-up observation, two factors related to low risk of breast cancer (multiparity and ovariectomy) were no longer so related. The most interesting finding is the increased risk of cancer among women with histories of histologically *confirmed benign breast disease*. The risk of breast cancer for women with benign breast disease diagnosed before estrogen use is about twice that of the general population. The risk among women with disease diagnosed after they started taking estrogen is *seven* times greater than that among the general population. These results emphasize the role of an estrogenic stimulus in the development of both benign and malignant breast disease. Moreover, they attest the relationship between benign and malignant breast lesions. All reports concerning the incidence of breast cancer in postmenopausal women using estrogen fail to give any indication of a possible association of progestins with the estrogen regimen.

2. *In the light of these results,* it seems reasonable to be very cautious in the management of hormone administration in postmenopausal women. Since the use of estrogen replacement in the menopause can provide real psychological and physical benefits to patients, it is clearly necessary to evaluate and treat the needs of patients individually. Possible additive risks, such as family history of breast cancer, or a long history of *untreated benign breast disease,* should be weighed as a contraindication to estrogen use. In other women, estrogen-replacement therapy should be given only in the case where estrogen deprivation is proven biologically, in particular by eliminating a possible extragonadal source of estrogen (for instance, peripheral conversion of androgen to estrone). In addition, it seems very reasonable to administer only low doses of estrogen associated with progestins given in a sequential mode with a view to reproducing the cyclicity in estrogen and progesterone production that depends on ovulation and adequate corpus luteum function.[31]

6. Conclusions

Benign breast diseases remain difficult to define from a clinical and pathological point of view. However, the progress realized in hormonal investigation—particularly the measurement of plasma steroids with accurate methods and the detection of steroid receptors in breast tissue—has yielded valuable information. These data lead to the conclusion that the different clinical expressions of these diseases are due to endocrine abnormalities. Indeed, benign breast diseases appear to be hormone-dependent at least at the beginning of their evolution. It seems reasonable to consider that they are induced by a hormonal environment characterized by an unopposed estrogen effect mainly due to an inadequate luteal function.

In addition, the presence *in vitro* of estradiol and progesterone receptors in lesions where the epithelial cells proliferate gives additional support to such a hypothesis.

Thus, recent lesions may be treated by the administration of progesterone and progestins to correct the systemic and local hormonal insufficiencies.

There is no proof that the same hormonal environment plays a major role in the development of breast cancer. There is only indirect evidence that favors a pathophysiological interpretation of human breast cancer epidemiology in terms of luteal insufficiency. However, it is obvious that there is no danger in considering the lack of progesterone secretion as a common risk factor for development of both benign breast diseases and cancer. The side effects resulting from treatment with progesterone and progestins are minor if not negligible. It is only by the early and long-continued treatment of a large cohort of patients, either with benign breast diseases or with high risk of developing breast cancer, that an answer may be given to such a speculation.

7. References

1. L. J. Humphrey, N. C. Estes, P. A. Morse, W. R. Jewel, R. A. Boudet, M. J. K. Hudson, P. G. Tsolakidis, and F. A. Mantz, Serum antibody in patients with breast disease: Correlation with histopathology, *Ann. Surg.* **180**, 124–129 (1974).
2. H. Davis, M. Simons, and J. B. Davis, Cystic disease of the breast: Relationship to carcinoma, *Cancer* **17**, 957–978 (1964).
3. C. D. Haagensen, *Diseases of the Breast*, W. B. Saunders, Philadelphia (1971).
4. P. K. Donnelly, K. W. Baker, J. A. Carney, and W. M. O'Fallon, Benign breast lesions and subsequent breast carcinoma in Rochester, Minnesota, *Mayo Clin. Proc.* **50**, 650–656 (1975).
5. R. V. Lloyd, Studies on the progesterone receptor content and steroid metabolism in normal and pathological human breast tissues, *J. Clin. Endocrinol. Metab.* **48**, 585–593 (1979).
6. J. De Brux, Histoire naturelle et diagnostic de quelques lésions mammaires, *Rev. Fr. Gynecol.* **68**, 365–388 (1973).
7. S. R. Wellings, H. M. Jensen, and R. G. Marcum, An atlas of subgross pathology of the human breast with special reference to possible precancerous lesions, *J. Natl. Cancer Inst.* **55**, 231–273 (1975).
8. R. Bässler, Morphology of hormone induced structural changes in the female breast, *Curr. Top. Pathol.* **53**, 1–89 (1970).
9. G. Asboe-Hansen, Hormonal effects on connective tissue, *Physiol. Rev.* **38**, 446–462 (1958).
10. H. Speert, "Pale epithelium" in the mammary gland and its experimental production in the rhesus monkey, *Surg. Gynecol. Obstet.* **74**, 1098–1106 (1942).
11. E. R. Fisher, Pathology of breast cancer, in: *Breast Cancer: Advances in Research and Treatment*, Vol. 1 (W. L. McGuire, ed.), pp. 43–123, Plenum Press, New York (1977).
12. M. Swerdlow and L. J. Humphrey, Fibrocystic disease and carcinoma of the breast, *Arch. Surg.* **87**, 457–460 (1963).
13. F. W. Foote, Jr., and F. W. Stewart, Comparative studies of cancerous versus non-cancerous breasts. II. Role of so-called chronic mastitis in mammary carcinogenesis, influence of certain hormones on human breast structure, *Ann. Surg.* **121**, 197–222 (1945).
14. L. J. Humphrey and M. Swerdlow, Relationship of benign breast disease to carcinoma of the breast, *Surgery* **52**, 841–846 (1962).
15. M. M. Black, T. H. C. Barclay, S. J. Cutler, B. F. Hankey, and A. J. Asire, Association of atypical characteristics of benign breast lesions with subsequent risk of breast cancer, *Cancer* **29**, 338–343 (1972).
16. H. Nagasawa, Prolactin and human breast cancer: A review, *Eur. J. Cancer* **15**, 267–279 (1979).
17. W. L. McGuire, G. C. Chamness, M. E. Costlow, and R. Shepherd, Hormone dependence in breast cancer, *Metabolism* **23**, 75–100 (1974).
18. W. L. McGuire, G. C. Chamness, M. E. Costlow, and N. Richert, Steroids and human breast cancer, *J. Steroid Biochem.* **6**, 723–728 (1975).

19. R. Sitruk-Ware, N. Sterkers, and P. Mauvais-Jarvis, Benign breast disease. I. Hormonal investigation, *Obstet. Gynecol.* **53**, 457–460 (1979).

20. W. L. McGuire, P. P. Carbone, and E. R. Vollmer, *Estrogen Receptors in Human Breast Cancer*, Raven Press, New York (1975).

21. W. L. McGuire, J. P. Raynaud, and E. E. Baulieu, *Progesterone Receptors in Normal and Neoplastic Tissues*, Raven Press, New York (1977).

22. P. Mauvais-Jarvis and F. Kuttenn, Les mastopathies bénignes, *Nouv. Presse Med.* **3**, 993–994 (1974).

23. H. Vorherr and R. H. Messer, Breast cancer: Potentially predisposing and protecting factors: Role of pregnancy, lactation and endocrine status, *Am. J. Obstet. Gynecol.* **130**, 335–358 (1978).

24. L. Tseng, S. B. Gusberg, and E. Gurpide, Estradiol receptor and 17β-dehydrogenase in normal and abnormal human endometrium, *Ann. N. Y. Acad. Sci.* **286**, 190–198 (1977).

25. A. J. W. Hsueh, E. J. Peck, and J. H. Clark, Control of uterine estrogen receptor levels by progesterone, *Endocrinology* **98**, 438–444 (1976).

26. J. C. Porter, Hormonal regulation of breast development and activity, *J. Invest. Dermatol.* **63**, 85–92 (1974).

27. D. Jacobsohn, Hormonal regulation of mammary gland growth, milk, in: *The Mammary Gland and Its Secretion* (S. K. Kon and A. T. Cowie, eds.), pp. 127–160, Academic Press, New York (1961).

28. A. T. Cowie, S. J. Folley, F. H. Malpress, and K. C. Richardson, Studies on the hormonal induction of mammary growth and lactation in the goat, *J. Endocrinol.* **8**, 64–88 (1952).

29. W. R. Lyons and D. A. McGinty, Effects of estrone and progesterone on male rabbit mammary glands. I. Varying doses of progesterone, *Proc. Soc. Exp. Biol. Med.* **48**, 83–89 (1941).

30. R. Sitruk-Ware, N. Sterkers, I. Mowszowicz, and P. Mauvais-Jarvis, Inadequate corpus luteum function in women with benign breast diseases, *J. Clin. Endocrinol. Metab.* **44**, 771–774 (1977).

31. P. Mauvais-Jarvis, F. Kuttenn, I. Mowszowicz, and R. Sitruk-Ware, Mastopathies bénignes: Etude hormonale chez 125 malades, *Nouv. Presse Med.* **6**, 4115–4118 (1977).

32. G. E. Abraham, G. B. Maroulis, and J. R. Marshall, Evaluation of ovulation and corpus luteum function using measurements of plasma progesterone, *Obstet. Gynecol.* **44**, 522–525 (1974).

33. E. V. Jensen, G. E. Block, S. Smith, K. Kyser, and E. R. Desombre, Estrogen receptors and breast cancer response to adrenalectomy: Predictor of response in cancer therapy, *Natl. Cancer Inst. Monogr.* **34**, 55–70 (1971).

34. S. G. Korenman and B. A. Dukes, Specific estrogen binding by the cytoplasm of human breast carcinoma, *J. Clin. Endocrinol. Metab.* **30**, 639–645 (1970).

35. G. Leclercq, J. C. Heuson, C. Deboel, and W. H. Mattheiem, Oestrogen receptors in breast cancer: A changing concept, *Br. Med. J.* **1**, 185–189 (1975).

36. B. S. Leung, L. C. Manaugh, and D. C. Wood, Estradiol receptors in benign and malignant disease of the breast, *Clin. Chim. Acta* **46**, 69–76 (1973).

37. P. P. Rosen, C. J. Menendez-Botet, J. S. Nisselbaum, J. A. Urban, V. Miké, A. Fracchia, and M. K. Schwartz, Pathological review of breast lesions analyzed for estrogen receptor protein, *Cancer Res.* **35**, 3187–3194 (1975).

38. P. Martin, F. Kuttenn, H. Serment, and P. Mauvais-Jarvis, Studies on clinical, hormonal and pathological correlations in breast fibroadenomas, *J. Steroid Biochem.* **9**, 1251–1256 (1978).

39. P. Martin, F. Kuttenn, H. Serment, and P. Mauvais-Jarvis, Progesterone receptors in breast fibroadenomas, *J. Steroid Biochem.* **11**, 1295–1298 (1979).

40. V. Cortes-Gallegos, A. J. Gallegos, C. S. Basurto, and J. Rivadeneyra, Estrogen peripheral levels vs estrogen tissue concentration in the human female reproductive tract, *J. Steroid Biochem.* **6**, 15–20 (1975).

41. R. Sitruk-Ware, B. Seradour, and C. Lafaye, Treatment of benign breast diseases by progesterone applied topically, in: *Percutaneous Absorption of Steroids* (P. Mauvais-Jarvis, C. H. F. Vickers, and J. Wepierre, eds.), pp. 219–229, Academic Press, London (1980).

42. N. Sterkers and J. Beauvais, Therapeutique progestative des mastodynies et mastopathies bénignes, *Senologia* **1**, 75 (1976).

43. P. Mauvais-Jarvis, N. Baudot, and J. P. Bercovici, *In vivo* studies on progesterone metabolism by human skin, *J. Clin. Endocrinol. Metab.* **29**, 1580–1585 (1969).

44. J. de Boever, B. Desmet, and D. Vandekerckhove, Variation of progesterone and estradiol concentrations in human mammary tissue and blood after topical administration of progesterone, in: *Percutaneous Absorption of Steroids* (P. Mauvais-Jarvis, C. H. F. Vickers, and J. Wepierre, eds.), pp. 259–265, Academic Press, London (1980).

45. M. Mori, T. Tominaga, and B. I. Tamaoki, Steroid metabolism in the normal mammary gland and in the dimethylbenzanthracene-induced mammary tumor of rats, *Endocrinology* **102**, 1387–1397 (1978).

46. P. Mauvais-Jarvis, N. Sterkers, F. Kuttenn, and J. Beauvais, Traitement des mastopathies bénignes par la progestérone et les progestatifs, *J. Gynecol. Obstet. Biol. Reprod. (Paris)* **7**, 477–484 (1978).

47. F. Kuttenn, A. Mouffarege, and P. Mauvais-Jarvis, Bases hormonales de la contraception progestative discontinue, *Nouv. Presse Med.* **7**, 3109–3113 (1978).

48. R. H. Asch and R. B. Greenblatt, The use of an impeded androgen—Danazol—in the management of benign breast disorders, *Am. J. Obstet. Gynecol.* **127**, 130–134 (1977).

49. W. P. Dmowski, Endocrine properties and clinical application of Danazol, *Fertil. Steril.* **31**, 237–251 (1979).

50. N. H. Lauersen and K. H. Wilson, The effect of Danazol in the treatment of chronic cystic mastitis, *Obstet. Gynecol.* **48**, 93–98 (1978).

51. R. H. Asch, E. O. Fernandez, C. G. Smith, T. M. Siler-Khodr, and C. J. Pauerstein, Effects of Danazol on gonadotropin levels in castrated rhesus monkeys, *Obstet. Gynecol.* **53**, 415–421 (1979).

52. N. H. Lauersen and K. H. Wilson, Danazol, an antigonadotropin agent in the treatment of pelvic endometriosis and chronic cystic mastitis, *Fertil. Steril.* **26**, 193 (1975).

53. N. H. Lauersen and K. H. Wilson, Evaluation of Danazol as an oral contraceptive, *Obstet. Gynecol.* **50**, 91–96 (1977).

54. B. K. Tsang, K. M. Henderson, and D. T. Armstrong, Effect of Danazol on estradiol-17β and progesterone secretion by porcine ovarian cells *in vitro*, *Am. J. Obstet. Gynecol.* **133**, 256–259 (1979).

55. B. M. Sherman and S. G. Korenman, Measurement of serum LH, FSH, estradiol and progesterone in disorders of the menstrual cycle: The inadequate luteal phase, *J. Clin. Endocrinol. Metab.* **39**, 145–149 (1974).

56. T. Backström and H. Cartensen, Estrogen and progesterone in plasma in relation to premenstrual tension, *J. Steroid Biochem.* **5**, 257–260 (1974).

57. T. Backström, L. Wide, R. Sodergard, and H. Cartensen, FSH, LH, TeBG capacity, estrogen and progesterone in women with premenstrual tension during the luteal phase, *J. Steroid Biochem.* **7**, 473–476 (1976).

58. G. E. Abraham, W. D. Odell, R. S. Swerdloff, and K. Hopper, Simultaneous radio immunoassay of plasma FSH, LH, progesterone, 17-hydroxyprogesterone and estradiol-17-β during the menstrual cycle, *J. Clin. Endocrinol. Metab.* **34**, 313–318 (1972).

59. H. Askalani, P, Wilkin, and J. Schwers, Serum progesterone in non pregnant women. II. Correlation between some progesterone and some other luteinization parameters, *Am. J. Obstet. Gynecol.* **118**, 1064–1069 (1974).

60. P. Mauvais-Jarvis and F. Kuttenn, Affections en rapport avec une anomalie de l'ovulation (anovulation et dysovulation), *Encycl. Med. Chir.* (Paris), Glandes Endocrines 10027 C¹⁰ (1974).

61. G. S. Richarson, Endometrial cancer as an estrogen progesterone target, *N. Engl. J. Med.* **286**, 645–647 (1972).

62. B. M. Sherman and S. G. Korenman, Hormonal characteristics of the human menstrual cycle throughout reproductive life, *J. Clin. Invest.* **55**, 699–706 (1975).

63. S. Matsumoto, M. Igarashi, and Y. Nagaoka, Environmental anovulatory cycles, *Int. J. Fertil.* **13**, 15–23 (1968).

64. G. C. L. Lachelin and S. S. C. Yen, Hypothalamic chronic anovulation, *Am. J. Obstet. Gynecol.* **130**, 825–831 (1978).

65. R. Grattarola, The premenstrual endometrial pattern of women with breast cancer, *Cancer* **17**, 1119–1122 (1964).

66. R. Grattarola, Androgens in breast cancer. I. Atypical endometrial hyperplasia and breast cancer in married premenopausal women, *Am. J. Obstet. Gynecol.* **116**, 423–428 (1973).

67. R. Grattarola, Anovulation and increased androgenic activity as breast cancer risk in woemn with fibrocystic disease of the breast, *Cancer Res.* **38**, 3051–3054 (1978).

68. P. Mauvais-Jarvis, G. Charransol, and F. Bobas-Masson, Simultaneous determination of urinary androstanediol and testosterone as an evaluation of human androgenicity, *J. Clin. Endocrinol. Metab.* **6**, 452–459 (1973).

69. R. Grattarola, The hormonal background of breast non cancerous diseases, *Senologia* **2**, 19–22 (1977).

70. F. Kuttenn, I. Mowszowicz, G. Schaison, and P. Mauvais-Jarvis, Androgen production and skin metabolism in hirsutism, *J. Endocrinol.* **75**, 83–91 (1977).

71. P. Mauvais-Jarvis, P. Lecomte, F. Kuttenn, I. Mowszowicz, J. Mandelbaum, and F. Gauthier-Wright, Etude hormonale complète de 12 cas d'ovaires polykystiques type (I), *Ann. Endocrinol.* **39**, 191–199 (1978).

72. B. MacMahon, P. Cole, and J. Brown, Etiology of human breast cancer: A review, *J. Natl. Cancer Inst.* **50**, 21–42 (1973).

73. R. D. Bulbrook, J. W. Moore, G. M. G. Clark, D. Y. Wang, D. Tong, and J. L. Hayward, Plasma oestradiol and progesterone levels in women with varying degrees of risk of breast cancer, *Eur. J. Cancer* **14**, 1369–1375 (1978).

74. F. de Waard, E. A. Baanders-Van Halewijn, and J. Huizinga, The bimodal age distribution of patients with mammary carcinoma, *Cancer* **17**, 141–151 (1964).

75. P. K. Siiteri and P. C. MacDonald, Role of extraglandular estrogen in human endocrinology, in: *Handbook of Physiology*, Vol. 2 (R. O. Greep and E. B. Astwood, eds.), pp. 615–629, American Physiological Society, Washington, D.C. (1973).

76. R. Hoover, L. A. Gray, P. Cole, and B. MacMahon, Menopausal estrogens and breast cancer, *N. Engl. J. Med.* **295**, 401–405 (1976).

77. B. M. Sherman and S. G. Korenman, Inadequate corpus luteum function: A pathophysiological interpretation of human breast cancer epidemiology, *Cancer* **33**, 1306–1312 (1974).

78. P. Mauvais-Jarvis, R. Sitruk-Ware, F. Kuttenn, and N. Sterkers, Luteal phase insufficiency: A common pathophysiological factor in development of benign and malignant breast diseases, in: *Commentaries on Research in Breast Disease* (R. D. Bulbrook and D. J. Taylor, eds.), pp. 25–59, Alan R. Liss, New York (1979).

79. R. E. Fechner, Fibrocystic disease in women receiving oral contraceptive hormones, *Cancer* **34**, 444–452 (1970).

80. F. G. Arthes, P. E. Sartwell, and E. F. Lewison, The pill, estrogens and the breast: Epidemiological aspects, *Cancer* **28**, 1391–1394 (1971).

81. M. R. Vessey, R. Doll, and R. Jones, Oral contraceptives and breast cancer: Progress report of an epidemiological study, *Lancet* **1**, 941–944 (1975).

82. H. Ory, P. Cole, B. MacMahon, and R. Hoover, Oral contraceptives and reduced risk of benign breast diseases, *N. Engl. J. Med.* **294**, 419–422 (1976).

83. A. Nomura and G. W. Comstock, Benign breast tumor and estrogenic hormones: A population-based retrospective study, *Am. J. Epidemiol.* **103**, 439–444 (1976).

84. M. P. Vessey, R. Doll, and P. M. Sutton, Oral contraceptives and breast neoplasia: A retrospective study, *Br. Med. J.* **3**, 719–724 (1972).

85. R. S. Paffenbarger, E. Fasal, M. E. Simmons, and J. B. Kampert, Cancer risk as related to use of oral contraceptives during fertile years, *Cancer* **39**, 1887–1891 (1977).

86. A. W. Lees, P. E. Burns, and M. Grace, Oral contraceptives and breast disease in premenopausal North Albertan women, *Int. J. Cancer* **22**, 700–707 (1978).

87. L. A. Brinton, R. R. Williams, R. N. Hoover, N. L. Stegens, M. Feinleib, and J. F. Fraumeni, Jr., Breast cancer risk factors among screening program participants, *J. Natl. Cancer Inst.* **62**, 37–44 (1979).

88. V. A. LiVolsi, B. V. Stadel, J. L. Kelsey, T. R. Holford, and C. White, Fibrocystic breast disease in oral contraceptive users: A histopathological evaluation of epithelial atypia, *N. Engl. J. Med.* **299**, 381–385 (1978).

89. Royal College of General Practitioners, Oral contraception study: Effect on hypertension and benign breast disease of progestagen component in combined oral contraceptives, *Lancet* **1**, 624 (1977).

90. R. A. Edgren and F. M. Sturtevant, Potencies of oral contraceptives, *Am. J. Obstet. Gynecol.* **125**, 1029–1038 (1976).

91. K. J. Ryan, Cancer risk and estrogen use in menopause, *N. Engl. J. Med.* **293**, 1199–1201 (1975).

92. J. Casagrande, V. Gerkins, B. E. Henderson, T. Mack, and M. C. Pike, Exogenous estrogens and breast cancer in women with natural menopause, *J. Natl. Cancer Inst.* **65**, 839–841 (1976).

93. J. Teter, Changing concepts in estrogen replacement therapy, Paper presented at the International Congress on the Menopause, La Grande Motte, France, June 8–10, p. 34 (1976).

94. L. E. Gerschenson, E. Conner, and J. T. Murai, Regulation of the cell cycle by diethylstilbestrol and progesterone in cultured endometrial cells, *Endocrinology* **100**, 1468–1471 (1977).

95. M. J. Eisen, The occurrence of benign and malignant mammary lesions in rats treated with crystalline estrogen, *Cancer Res.* **2**, 632–644 (1942).

96. A. E. Treloar, R. E. Boynton, B. G. Behn, and B. W. Brown, Variation of the human menstrual cycle through reproductive life, *Int. J. Fertil.* **12**, 77–126 (1967).

97. P. Mauvais-Jarvis and F. Kuttenn, L'insuffisance en progestérone est-elle cancérigène?, *Nouv. Presse Med.* **4**, 323–326 (1975).

98. P. F. A. Van Look, W. M. Hunter, I. S. Fraser, and D. T. Baird, Impaired estrogen induced luteinizing hormone release in young women with anovulatory dysfunctional uterine bleeding, *J. Clin. Endocrinol. Metab.* **46**, 816–823 (1978).

4

A Patient Looks at Breast Cancer at the Beginning of a New Decade

ROSE KUSHNER

1. Prologue

A patient writing a chapter about breast cancer in a medical text for scientists is faced with a dilemma: she does not and cannot see the picture as seen by the eyes of an investigator or a clinician. Nor can they see hers.

There may be pathologists and biologists who have studied breast cancer for years but who have never had the chance to talk to a woman who has this disease. To them, mammary carcinoma may involve the bizarre behavior of a bizarre collection of cells that they watch *in vitro, in vivo,* or under the microscope.

Clinicians—be they surgical or medical oncologists—do get to know the patient, but they are frequently so intent on the disease itself that they do not understand what she is thinking about.

Nowhere is the dicohotomy between patient and scientist so evident as it is when the patient has been asked to write a chapter for the scientist to read, even if the information has nothing to do with the emotional aspects of breast cancer.

An excellent example of these differing views is evident in the arrangement of the subject matter in this patient-written chapter in comparison with the way the same material was presented in the earlier volumes of *Breast Cancer: Advances in Research and Treatment.*

Histology—its mysteries of *in situ* lesions, preneoplasia, hyperplasia, dysplasia, anaplasia, metaplasia; stromal, lymphatic, and

ROSE KUSHNER • Breast Cancer Advisory Center, Kensington, Maryland 20795. ©1979, 1980.

blood-vessel invasion; nuclear typing and nuclear grading—are all incorporated into Vol. 1 of the series, *Current Approaches to Therapy*. But in this chapter, these issues are discussed within the framework of the biology of breast cancer.

Why?

Because women are concerned with how much of their bodies must be lost in order to be rid of the disease. Since women cannot be put in laboratory cages to be inoculated with a virus, chemical, or hormone, the only way to study human breast-cancer biology is by analyzing the long-term results of various approaches to breast-cancer therapy.

Along the same lines, biological, biochemical, immunological, and histological "markers" are considered, by a patient, to be procedures for detection—"prognostic indicators."

Why?

Because it is hoped that all of them will, some day, be able to detect the presence or absence of cancer in her body. As such indicators, these topics would be included in Vol. 3, *Current Topics*, along with mammography—not in *Experimental Biology*.

On the other hand, etiology and epidemiology—subjects that are discussed in Vol. 3—would be included in *Experimental Biology* where the roles of hormones, viruses, and genetics in the cause of breast cancer are described. To women, epidemiology means who? where? and when?—and the answers would be populations at high risk.

Patients have a totally different view of the various scientific approaches, and reading the work described in *Breast Cancer* does give a patient a better understanding of the way the disease appears from the vantage point of the laboratory and clinic. It is hoped that the reverse will also be true.

The Breast Cancer Advisory Center was founded in September 1975 to respond to anticipated letters and telephone calls resulting from the publication of my book, *Breast Cancer; A Personal History & an Investigative Report*. Established as a "temporary" source of information, the center has helped more than 10,000 women (and men) deal with problems regarding every aspect of breast cancer—from what a high-risk teen-ager can do to legal action to fight job and credit discrimination. The center is a nonprofit health service organization and is funded entirely by voluntary contributions from individuals, health groups, and business firms.

2. Introduction

In 1971, the Congress of the United States passed the National Cancer Act and created the National Cancer Program (NCP). This event heralded the beginning of a decade of unparalleled progress in the basic research, detection, diagnosis, and treatment of all cancers. In the case of breast cancer, the developments of the next ten years came so rapidly that it was difficult to write a brochure, pamphlet, article, or book that would not become obsolete before it saw the dark of print.

This was not the case before the NCP began. Despite intensive research all over the world during the preceding century, survival rates of women who developed breast cancer had not changed since the 1930s.[1] The National Cancer Institute (NCI)—established in 1937—had made much progress in the prevention, detection, diagnosis, and treatment of other malignant diseases, but breast-cancer statistics remained grim.

It was hoped that the NCP would alter the situation. Having sent men to the moon in 1969, the Congress believed the same kind of concentrated, multidisciplinary effort would eradicate cancer by the country's 200th birthday—the Bicentennial Year.[2] The goal was considered unrealistic by virtually all members of the scientific community involved in cancer research at that time. These people knew that more than sophisticated technology was needed to unravel the mysteries of this bizarre collection of invasive diseases in a mere five years. So passage of the act was received with mixed feelings: many people believed that failure to achieve the goal set by Congress would jeopardize long-range programs the NCI had already launched.[3]

For example, before the NCP began, women (and men) who developed breast cancer were already benefiting from NCI research. In 1957, the National Surgical Adjuvant Breast Project (NSABP) had been created, and in 1966, Congress had authorized the formation of the Breast Cancer Task Force (BCTF). After the act was signed, the NSABP was incorporated into the Treatment Committee of the BCTF, and by October 1970, all related disciplines were united under the aegis of the BCTF—a single committee mobilized to fight breast cancer.[4] Medical oncology, program-planning, biometrics, biochemistry, virology, surgery, pathology, and radiation therapy were all represented.

When the BCTF evaluated "the state of the art" at the beginning of 1970, it found many schools of thought about all aspects of breast cancer, but data—except for those of the NSABP—were based on such small samples that firm criteria, acceptable to everyone, could not be established.[5]

By 1980, there are still different schools of thought about most aspects of breast-cancer detection, diagnosis, and treatment. Data in some areas are still relatively helter-skelter, but these areas are new ones—unheard of in 1970. Are progesterone receptors important? Is a medical adrenalectomy as good as one achieved with the scalpel? When should a woman under age 50 be mammographed? For the 1970 problems, the samples are larger; for these modern-day quandaries, there is the old, familiar refrain: the numbers are too small to be statistically significant.

To show how much has happened in the past decade, from the patient's point of view, this chapter is divided into two sections: "The 'State of the Art' in 1970" and "The 'State of the Art' in 1980." Perspectives may differ, but the magnitude of the ten years' accomplishments is on the record for all to see.

3. The "State of the Art" in 1970

3.1. Biology

The National Cancer Institute (NCI) and research laboratories all over the world had been studying the transformation of healthy cells to malignant ones for decades. Advanced technologies enabled scientists to learn how cells function in detail that was never possible before, and the body of knowledge accumulated about all cancer contributed to a greater understanding of this complex group of diseases. The fact that there were more than a hundred types of "cancer"—all different from one another—was the inevitable outcome of this research. It was obvious that there could be no one "cure" for all of them.

In the case of breast cancer, it was known that there are at least 15 variations of this disease, each having its own "doubling time" or speed of mitotic activity. Thus, there could be relatively "benign" cancers that invaded slowly and others that were aggressive and virulent. Gershon-Cohen et al.[6] had reported that the fastest-growing tumor cells doubled every 23 days; the slowest, every 209 days. This meant that a lesion weighing a gram and containing an estimated billion cells had been growing in the breast for about two years. This knowledge about cell kinetics became increasingly important to women who developed the disease, because it supported the idea of detecting potential tumors when they were nonpalpable. Chemotherapy—its dose and schedule of administration—also depends on estimates of cell kill to be effective.

Thanks to the work of the NSABP, additional knowledge had been amassed about the biology of breast cancer, especially of metastasis. This knowledge of the result of years of large-scale clinical trials involved the cooperation of 45 institutions. Beginning in the late 1950's, they had begun studies of both recurrence and survival rates of breast-cancer patients who had been treated by radical mastectomy.[7] When 5-year rates were analyzed, the results showed that neither recurrence nor survival depended on the size of the primary tumor—as had always been believed—but on the number of positive axillary lymph nodes found at the time of surgery.

Even when the lesion was as small as 1.0 cm, if more than four axillary nodes were positive, 5-year recurrences were high; survival rates were low. Conversely, women with 3.0-cm tumors whose axillary nodes were free of cancer had lower rates of recurrence and better survivals.[8]

Fisher and Fisher[9] concluded that the dissemination of breast cancer was not always the result of direct invasion from tissue to tissue, but could be the result of blood- or lymph-borne emboli that infiltrated the body by numerous routes, regardless of the tumor's size. If this were true, the disease was probably systemic from its inception. In such cases, extensive surgical procedures would make no difference in the ultimate outcomes.[9]

Subsequent NSABP studies showed that the disease—even when it spread via the axillary nodes—was not orderly, from node to node.[10] Nor did cancer cells always succeed in implanting the disease to other parts of the body: there was strong evidence of immune resistance by the host, a reaction that interfered with metastasis.[11]

Of course, to women, the data concerning extensive surgery were the most important biological findings; to scientists, the absence of a constant correlation between the size of a patient's tumor and the stage of her disease was more significant, because "small" had always meant "early" and "large" had always meant late. Because of these results, the stage was set for massive breast-screening programs designed to detect the disease in its nonpalpable, subclinical stage. These programs, the Breast Cancer Detection Demonstration Projects (BCDDPs), were launched in 1972 with the joint sponsorship of the NCI and the American Cancer Society (ASC).

3.2. Etiology and Epidemiology

Little is known in 1980 about the causes of breast cancer, and still less was known a decade ago. In 1970, patients interested in the esoteric aspects of the cause and spread of breast cancer would have learned that female hormones—estrogens—had long been implicated. Ever since 1896, when Beatson[12] discovered that women frequently improved if their ovaries were removed, scientists had been pursuing estrogens for both cause and cure.[13]

The role of a virus in the etiology of breast cancer was suspected to be important.[14] Bittner[15] had proven that breast cancer was transmitted via lactation in mice, and there was proof that other cancers could grow after transplantation from one animal to another.[16]

Among lay people, the knowledge that breast cancer "runs in the family" seemed to support the viral theory, and the disease was often believed to be contagious. Although there was mounting evidence that a dot of DNA, not a transmissible virus, was the chief culprit, human breast-cancer cells, at that time, died *in vitro* after about 30 passages. Therefore, neither theory could be studied adequately, because virtually all such research depended on animal models.

By the end of the 1960's, data from the Biological Effects of Ionizing Radiation Commission were indicating that the atomic-bomb survivors in Hiroshima and Nagasaki had developed breast cancer in excess of the normal Japanese incidence.[17,17a] Although some chemicals were carcinogenic (for breast cancer) in animals, as far as anyone knew, none was present in any food or substance in ordinary use.[18] Exogenous estrogens had been marketed for contraception since 1960, and opposition to "loading" the systems of young women with extra hormones was developing.[19] However, because estrogenic postmenopausal medications had been available since the 1940's, with no evidence, at that time, associating these steroids with breast cancer, "the pill" was considered safe.[20]

Epidemiology was an infant science that showed promise for identifying high-risk subgroups of women, and it was apparent that knowing more about them would yield information about the etiology of the disease.[21] For example, MacMahon and Cole had studied large populations of breast-cancer patients and had shown that many factors appeared to be involved.

Women who had already had breast cancer were at highest risk of developing another; daughters and sisters of breast-cancer patients—especially if the patients had had premenopausal bilateral disease—were also at high risk. If a woman had a personal history of benign breast disease, her chances of developing a malignant one increased.

The length of a woman's reproductive life, or more specifically, how old she was at menarche and menopause, affected relative risk: early onset of menstruation and its late cessation were associated with higher incidences; late onset and early menopause (natural or artificial) were correlated with lower risks. Women who had never borne living children appeared to have an excess of breast cancer. Conversely, women who delivered their first child prior to the age of 18 had lower risks.

Other factors included race, ethnic and religious ancestry, socioeconomic status, and total body volume, i.e., height and weight.[22]

3.3. Detection and Diagnosis

In 1970, women were usually not diagnosed to have breast cancer until the lesion was so advanced that axillary lymph nodes were positive in about 75% of cases.[23] The recommendation that women practice regular breast self-examination was being made by the ACS and the

NCI, but large-scale public-education programs about the practice were still in the early planning stages. However, a "new" diagnostic modality using X-ray was proving its usefulness.

Mammography was first introduced by Salomon[24] in 1913, and in the 1930s, Gershon-Cohen,[25] Egan,[26] and other radiologists urged that X-rays of the breast be used to screen women to detect breast lesions during their subclinical stage. In 1961, the Health Insurance Plan (HIP) of New York City began conducting randomized trials of 30,000 of its members, utilizing mammography. The purpose of the trials was to compare survival rates of those women whose cancers were discovered by X-ray plus clinical examination with those of members who had only clinical examination.[27]

Strax et al.[28] published the first 5-year results of the HIP study in 1969, and there was a one third decrease in the mortality rates of post-menopausal women. Since there had been considerable progress in radiological technology since the trial began, Strax and Holleb[29] believed that these advances would be reflected by an increase in the number of early cancers found in younger women. With this hope, the ACS planned 12 national demonstration projects in which women—self-selected and *not* randomized—would be screened annually for 5 years. The screening process was to include a clinical examination, mammography, and thermography—a technique that photographs the breast via infrared film to measure its heat-retention patterns.[30] Every women participating in the program was to be followed for 5 years after the screenings were terminated.[31]

The NSABP data relevant to the metastatic potential of even microscopic tumors convinced the Breast Cancer Task Force that this ACS program should be broadened and supported. Therefore, plans were then being made to establish 27 BCDDPs and each was to accrue 10,000 women. The goal of the projects, from the NCI point of view, would be, not to compare survival rates, but to see whether more than a quarter of a million women would volunteer to be screened. Thus, the BCDDP was not designed to be the kind of comparative, randomized, clinical trial the HIP study was.[32]

Although mammography and thermography dominated early-detection research in 1970, there was work being done to find a potential "Pap smear" for breast cancer by aspirating nipple fluid.[33] Ultrasonography seemed promising,[34] and immunologists had reported a variety of cell-surface antigens—in particular, carcinoembryonic antigen (CEA)—that might be "markers," in either blood or urine, signaling the presence of primary or metastatic disease.[35] Other components of blood and urine were also the subjects of considerable research. [36,37] A search for immunological factors in the tumor itself, factors that might aid in prognosis, was being conducted by several investigators, but data were sparse and too preliminary to be meaningful. [38-40]

Nuclear medicine, and its possible importance in detecting early distant metastases, was sometimes a routine part of a presurgical work-up, but this practice was not common. [41] Conventional X-rays were used to detect osseous recurrences *after* surgery, but—even if there was an effective technique for detecting micrometastases preoperatively—performing such examinations was not cost-effective. There was little to be done even if such asymptomatic metastatic lesions could be found. [42]

3.4. Primary Treatment

In 1970, a woman who found a possible symptom of breast cancer could expect to be admitted to a hospital for an overnight stay and given a general anesthetic for the diagnostic biopsy. Until she woke up in the recovery room, she would not know whether she still had two breasts or if one had been removed while she was asleep. At that time, the standard radical mastectomy (the Halsted) was still—after three fourths of a century—the most common surgical treatment for primary breast cancer in the United States. [43-45] This meant that women who found even the smallest tumor could expect to lose a breast, both their pectoral muscles, and their axillary lymph nodes. All too often, the surgery resulted in disfiguring defects that crippled women emotionally and in lymphedema that could affect their normal functioning. Not knowing in advance whether the breast would be lost seemed to make the word biopsy synonymous with radical mastectomy. [46]

Of course, this entire ordeal was already known to be unnecessary. As explained earlier, NSABP trials had shown that extensive dissection and resection did not affect ultimate survival: the same trial that proved tumor size to be unrelated to survival also proved that the extent of the surgery did not increase survival rates. If a woman's axillary nodes were negative, her chances of being alive 10 years after primary surgery were good; if she had one to three positive nodes, the odds fell; if more than four nodes contained metastasis, her prognosis was poor. [47]

Although all the women in this trial had been treated by a "radical mastectomy," there was little uniformity in terms of the precise details of the procedure performed. Some surgeons excised more tissue than others did; some removed both the pectoralis major and the pectoralis minor, while others preserved the latter. Varying numbers of axillary nodes were excised. When the results were analyzed, it was found that the primary surgery, i.e., the quantity of tissue removed, did not affect survival rates. [48]

Because of the outcome of this trial, the NSABP did not even consider evaluating the extended (or supraradical) mastectomy advocated by many surgeons here and abroad.[49,50] Instead, the next NSABP trial, regarding primary surgical treatment, would compare the Halsted radical mastectomy to even lesser procedures that preserved the breast and axillary nodes.[51,52]

Although women knew there were surgeons in this country and elsewhere who removed only the lesion in a "lumpectomy" or tylectomy, with and without irradiation, this procedure was not yet ready for clinical trials. The directors of the NSABP felt that its studies regarding the possible reduction of surgery should be orderly.[51,52]

On another front, a project-supported randomized trial, begun in 1961 and involving more than 300 women, demonstrated no significant differences in survivals of women who had had postmastectomy prophylactic oophorectomies and those who had not.[53] Another NSABP trial began in the same year to see whether postoperative irradiation of the axilla resulted in increased survival rates. According to Fisher, while the incidence of local and regional recurrences did decrease, there was no difference in survival rates between the two groups.[54]

All the NSABP trials proved conclusively that a woman's ultimate fate depends on the number of positive nodes found in her axilla at the time of mastectomy.[55] Although this "barometer" has been described as crude and primitive,[56] nodal status was (and still is) the only reliable prognostic indicator available.[57] In 1980, as in 1970, the end results of breast-cancer patients are correlated with the quantity of disease found beyond the breast.[58]

3.5. Adjuvant Therapy

In the 1950's, combinations of anticancer drugs were found to be effective against leukemia and Hodgkin's disease,[59] and their success prompted attempts to fight breast cancer in the same way. Until then, chemotherapy had been used to treat breast-cancer patients only when surgery, radiation, steroids, and other palliative measures failed to stop the metastatic spread. By 1958, chemotherapy had been successful enough in the treatment of metastatic disease that the time had come to try anticancer drugs prophylactically.

There was good reason to believe they would be effective. NSABP data showing that a large number of breast-cancer patients already had disseminated micrometastases at the time of diagnosis also suggested that these occult clusters of cells might be destroyed by systemic treatment administered immediately after surgery. Since nodal status was the only risk indicator known, the logical candidates for such "adjuvant chemotherapy" were those with positive axillary nodes.[60]

In 1958, the NSABP initiated a double-blind randomized trial to compare triethylenethiophosphoramide (thio-TEPA or TSPA) with a placebo, and the 5-year follow-up data of the trial were stratified by nodal as well as menopausal status. When these were analyzed, there was a 33% greater survival rate among the premenopausal women receiving TSPA who had had four or more positive axillary nodes than in any of the other subgroups.[61]

The next study compared 5-flourouracil (5-FU) with TSPA and a placebo. The women who were given 5-FU suffered from considerable toxicity, but they did not do as well as did the control group receiving the placebo. Women with four or more positive nodes who had been given TSPA had significantly lower recurrence rates at the end of 5 years.

While this trial might have seemed disappointing at the time, it did show that neither drug was beneficial as adjuvant therapy for postmenopausal women. More important, the success of adjuvant chemotherapy in the subgroup of premenopausal women was evidence that the principle of using prophylactic anticancer drugs—in high-risk women, before any signs of recurrence appeared—was indeed valid.

3.6. Metastatic Disease

Of course, the reason breast cancer is, too often, a fatal disease is that the treatment of an early, localized tumor may not be enough. The primary treatment—be it some type of radical mastectomy, lesser surgery, or radiation, alone or in combination—is, by definition, local therapy. By 1970, statistics had shown that about half of all women who developed breast cancer eventually died of their disease.[62] Because routine postmastectomy oophorectomy and local irradiation often did nothing to prolong life, much hope and money were being invested in the success of prophylactic adjuvant chemotherapy.[63] But these trials were just beginning in 1970, and women with existing recurrent or metastatic disease would not be helped by them.

The weapons in the oncologist's arsenal for treating disseminated disease included surgery, X-ray therapy, hormonal manipulation (additive or ablative), and chemotherapy—alone or in combination with other anticancer agents.

X-ray was the major nonsurgical modality used both for therapy, i.e., to bring about a regression, and for palliative relief of the pain of skeletal metastases.[64] As mentioned earlier, endocrine manipulation was widely used, and oophorectomy was usually the first treatment of choice for premenopausal women with recurrent or metastatic disease.

About one third of the time, this procedure resulted in complete remissions, although the disease-free interval rarely lasted longer than 18 months.[65]

When patients were older than 55 years of age, results of endocrine manipulation varied: both additive hormonal therapy with large doses of estrogens and—paradoxically—androgens appeared to help different populations of postmenopausal women.

It the metastases had responded to either oophorectomy or additive endocrine therapy by regression or remission, their reappearance was often treated surgically by bilateral adrenalectomy or hypophysectomy. These procedures sometimes brought about additional disease-free months, but their morbidity was high enough to cause physicians to be reluctant to perform the operations.[66]

Thio-TEPA, 5-FU, cytoxan, and a newly developed tumorcidal drug—adriamycin—were used as single agents or in combination with both surgical and medical endocrine manipulation. However, ultimately, the disease took over, and the only efforts to be made concerned control of the pain.

3.7. Psychosocial Aspects of Breast Cancer

In 1952, Terese Lasser, a woman who had undergone a radical mastectomy, decided that something should be done to help women cope with the physical and emotional problems associated with the loss of a breast. At that time, it was often impossible to find professionally made prostheses, brassieres, and clothing—especially bathing suits—designed to cover or disguise the defects left by the surgery. Most important, the excision of the axillary lympatics usually left women's affected arms impaired, swollen, and painful. [67]

Mrs. Lasser's organization provided much-needed personal support and information to new breast-cancer patients. With the surgeon's permission, volunteers, who had themselves had mastectomies, visited patients the hospital, gave them temporary prostheses, simple equipment to exercise the arm, and compiled lists of stores where permanent breast forms and suitable clothing were available. In 1968, the ACS incorporated the organization into its national rehabilitation program as "Reach to Recovery." The local unit of the ACS was frequently the only place a woman could go for help after having had a mastectomy.[46]

Bard and Sutherland[68] and Barckley[69] studied and wrote about the emotional problems following radical mastectomy, but little was done except to identify and recognize them. At that time, the quantity of a woman's life was the prime medical concern, and the quality of her remaining months or years seemed to be less important.[70]

As described earlier, women who developed possible symptoms of breast cancer could expect to be anesthetized for the diagnostic biopsy without knowing in advance whether or not their diagnoses would be positive or negative. Because little was generally known about the biology of breast cancer, it was thought that separating the diagnostic biopsy from definitive treatment would "seed" the cancer and speed its spread to other organs. As a result, any kind of presurgical counseling and emotional preparation was impossible.

For those women who awakened with both breasts, the postoperative period was filled with relief and happiness. Those who awoke to find that the breast had been removed faced more immediate problems than lost body image, sexuality, and femininity. Although there was considerable evidence that these concerns often outweighed their fear of the disease, little had been written and still less had been done to help them.[71]

Cronin *et al.* [72] had described possible techniques to rebuild the lost breast using plastic-surgery techniques, but the absence of suitable materials made the procedure difficult and, many believed, dangerous. However, inadequate technology was not the major obstacle. The initial surgery—the standard radical mastectomy—resulted in the loss of so much tissue that there was no muscle for anchoring an implant and thin skin flaps to cover it (if a good one had been developed at the time).

Of course, most women survived the emotional ordeal, but many did not. They lived as recluses and semiinvalids.[73] Except for the types of women who became active in organizations such as Reach to Recovery, those who had had mastectomies often kept the surgery a secret, even from their children and close relatives and friends. In 1970, breast cancer was still a "taboo" subject in the United States, almost in the same category as syphyllis and gonorrhea.[74]

4. The "State of the Art" in 1980

4.1. Biology

To women, biological knowledge gained by electron microscopy, radioimmunoassay, chromatography, DNA, RNA, reverse transcriptase, enzymes, isoenzymes, steroids, nucleotides, and other means is not meaningful. Of course, they realize that understanding the development of cancer is essential if either a prevention or a cure is ever to be found. But—to women—the most important aspect of its biology is those data showing that less surgery can be safely used as primary treatment. While the decade between 1970 and 1980 did produce a wealth of such evidence, an unexpected biological development occurred to reverse this trend: the concept that the presence of "preneoplasia" is a justification for surgery.

Wide acceptance of this concept is already creating problems for women (and the situation will undoubtedly continue or even worsen), and it is overshadowing the results of the past decade's research proving that less, not more, extensive primary surgery is necessary. For this reason, biological developments related to pathogenesis are most important, from a patient's point of view.

According to Gallager and Hutter,[75] the "inception" of a mammary carcinoma is an almost inevitable continuum, beginning with hyperplasia. They base this belief on animal models, because, in mice, hyperplastic alveolar nodules (HANs) are always precursors of the disease. However, not all the animals with HANs go on to develop invasive cancers.[76] Nonetheless, many scientists assume that an extrapolation can be made from mouse to woman, and the fact that having a history of benign breast disease increases the risk of developing breast cancer is used as evidence supporting it.[77-78]

Gallager and Martin[79] studied serial sections from cancer-containing breasts and found multiple preneoplastic lesions and true carcinomas in as many as 50% of them. As far as the contralateral breast is concerned, Gallager reports the development of multicentric foci in as many as 65% of cases. However, this has been contradicted by others.[80]

To women reading these data, the findings are bewildering. First of all, what can women having histories of benign breast disease do about their high risk of developing a future malignancy? Surely, scientists and practicing physicians should, by now, be able to do more than simply tell them to be alert and practice breast self-examination. Are there not certain characteristics—biochemical, histological, and immunological "markers"—that can be found on the premalignant, but still benign, lesion that can be analyzed to predict the woman's future fate?

Second, there is clear evidence from Gallager's own studies, as well as from those of others,[81] that not all atypia, in situ, or even true cancers grow to become life-threatening. Third, if and when this has been shown to happen in the ipsilateral or contralateral breast, many years—as many as 22—intervened. Some women, if given a choice, would opt to live those years with two breasts, despite the uncertainty about centricles. Logically, if multicentricity in the contralateral breast is so high, should both not be removed? Finally, if there is a 50% chance of having other malignant foci, there is also a 50% chance of *not* having any.

The complexity of the problem is compounded by the knowledge that older women, dead of other diseases, have been found to have undetected breast cancers on autopsy, cancers that never progressed to the stage where they became symptomatic.[82]

Breast-cancer biologists, pathologists, and surgeons, no doubt, view all these contradictory data abstractly. But a woman looking at the welter of conflicting opinions realizes that no one really knows what to do about these noncancerous "cancers." As a result, she must fear that many mastectomies are being performed to treat lesions that are never going to become fatal.

Until mammography became so widely used for diagnosis of early breast cancer, the question of what is temporarily preneoplastic and what is permanently hyperplastic was not important to women. Nor was another continuing argument important: does the disease remained localized for a finite period of time before becoming regional, then stay in the nodes for a specific interval before being disseminated as distant metastases? While scientists might have pondered these problems, their ponderings made no difference to women. The reason for this indifference was simple: if the lesion was too small to be detected manually, they did not know it was there. On the other hand, if its cells were invasive, this eventually became evident.

Mammography has changed this. The device is so exquisitely sensitive that it can detect microscopic spots that may be such preneoplastic or *in situ* clusters of cells. Finding such suspicious areas has become so commonplace that special techniques have been developed to identify them so surgeons can know where to put their scalpels,[83] and specimen radiography was invented to be sure the nonpalpable "lesion" had actually been excised.[84] For most surgeons, there is no problem. They consider these lesions to be "minimal" or "Stage 0" breast cancers that, if left untreated, would inevitably become invasive. They also believe the degree of multicentricity to be so high that an entire breast must be removed for even the smallest number of noninvasive cells. Therefore, a total mastectomy with, at least, an axillary sampling is the only cure.

However, women who read the asterisked small print at the bottom of most incidence tables can find the words, "Excluding skin cancer and carcinoma in situ of the cervix."[85] They cannot help but wonder why a carcinoma *in situ* of the cervix is not even considered to be cancer by statisticians, but the same minimal disease—when found in the breast—requires the extensive surgery used for large invasive cancers. Of course, saving her life is every woman's prime concern. But if she can accomplish this by less than having a mastectomy, this would certainly be her treatment of choice.

In the past, women considered research into the biological history of breast cancer to be somehow related to the work of counting the number of angels dancing on the head of a pin. But now, this area is of critical importance to women. Answers must be found to the following questions:

1. What kinds of lesions are truly preneoplastic?
2. What lesions will probably remain hyperplastic, anaplastic, metaplastic, or otherwise atypical for the rest of her life?
3. Which lesions are truly *in situ*, and which are not?
4. Exactly how multicentric is breast cancer?
5. Do different cell types have varying degrees of multicentricity?
6. If so, what kind of treatment is necessary for each?

These are the questions women want answered by breast-cancer biologists and pathologists.

The Breast Cancer Detection Demonstration Projects (BCDDPs) will contribute data that will help answer these questions within the next decade. Of the 280,000 women screened, about 15,000 were found to have suspicious lesions in their breasts, but biopsies were not performed. In addition, there were some women whose biopsies showed *in situ* or atypical diagnosis but who had either no further treatment or some type of segmental surgery. These participants in the BCDDPs are also being followed by the NCI, and their ultimate outcomes will yield important data.[86]

National Surgical Adjuvant Breast Project trials will, again, be a rich source of biological data. The first NSABP surgical clinical trial to compare primary treatment began in the fall of 1971. About 1700 women were examined clinically, and those with negative axillary nodes were randomized into three groups: radical mastectomy, total mastectomy with radiation of the axilla, and total mastectomy alone. Patients who subsequently developed positive axillary nodes (about 15%) had dissections.

By February 1981, there were no significant differences in the appearance of distant metastases or in the survival rates of patients in the three treatment groups. This study is biologically important, because about 40% of the women with clinically negative axillary nodes (randomized into the radical-mastectomy arm of the trial) were later found to have regional metastases histologically. Therefore, it is reasonable to assume that about 40% of the women in the other two groups had the same incidence. While radiation is a substitute for surgery, those women who had neither dissection nor X-ray have not suffered any higher rate of distant metastases or death from breast cancer than did the two treated groups.

Thus, this study is evidence that removing the axillary nodes is not a therapeutic procedure but a diagnostic one for staging the extent of the disease.[87]

Although these women are still being followed, there were enough data, in early 1976, to persuade the NSABP to design a protocol comparing even lesser surgical procedures. By April, the project began accruing patients for randomization into three groups: total mastectomy, segmental resection followed by radiation of the preserved breast, and segmental resection alone. Axillary dissections are done for staging. Unfortunately, accruing women into this protocol was difficult at the beginning, but by the end of February, 1981, about 860 had been randomized in the United States and Canada.

Another NCI-supported trial began in mid-1979 to evaluate two procedures: total mastectomy (followed by breast reconstruction) and local excision of the tumor with postoperative radiation of the intact breast and adjacent tissue, when necessary. Axillary dissections are also required for this protocol.

Of course, the results of both these clinical trials were too preliminary, by the end of 1979, to have yielded any useful data. For women, their end results will be vitally important, because—together with those from the BCDDPs—they may finally provide an answer to the question: is it always necessary to amputate the breast?

4.2. Etiology and Epidemiology

The decade that linked lung cancer to cigarette-smoking and certain liver cancers to vinyl chloride also produced new clues about the multiple causes of breast cancer. However, in 1980, these are still nothing but clues. The only carcinogen that has definitely been proven to cause human breast cancer is low-dose ionizing radiation.

Except for the fetus, the breast is the most radiosensitive of any human tissue,[88] but this was not known in the preceding decades. Early in the 1970s, the Biological Effects of Ionizing Radiation report described the high post war incidence in Japanese survivors and attributed the rise to fallout from the atomic raids. But not until the BCDDP crisis in 1976 (detailed later) was the question addressed. Then, retrospective studies indicated that women who had had multiple X-ray exposures developed high rates of the disease, and Upton et al.[89] showed that low-dose radiation could cause breast cancer.

Most etiological data have come from meticulous laboratory research and from large-scale epidemiological studies. For basic scientists, perhaps the most important event was the development of methodologies that permit a mammary gland and its tumor to be kept alive *in vitro* for generations, and the next momentous step was being able to do the same with cancer-cell lines.[90] By the end of 1979, countless human and lower-animal explants and at least 15 different strains of living cancer cells were in the world's laboratories.

Until these *in vitro* methodologies evolved, most laboratory research relied on animal models: on nude mice to eliminate any role of the host's immune system, on *in vivo* studies to learn the effects of various substances. With human tissue available, there is no longer a need to assume or to extrapolate. Progress in biomedical research, it seems, always follows advances in technology—be it the microscope or the microcomputer.

As stated earlier, hormones, specifically estrogens, have been empirically implicated with breast cancer for almost a century, but not until the work of Lacassagne,[91] beginning in 1932, were estrogens studied experimentally. Whether they are carcinogens, procarcinogens, or cocarcinogens[92] is still unknown, but Dao[93] evades this semantic problem by saying that a large proportion of both animal and human breast cancers "depends on estrogens to flourish."

Lemon[94] suspects only estrone and estradiol and considers estriol to be protective; Kirschner[95] has described a serum estrogen fraction—E_3/E_1+E_2—to be an important factor in providing a hospitable environment where a breast cancer (perhaps caused by something else) can grow. Whether progesterone enhances or inhibits growth of breast cancer is a source of scientific uncertainty.[96]

Lippman[97] sums the situation up nicely, for women, by simply stating that "... the effects of steroid hormones remain controversial."

To women, the "estrogen factor" is of special significance. Warnings issued by the Food & Drug Administration (FDA) against usage of both estrogenic oral contraceptives and estrogenic postmenopausal replacement medications by women who have had breast cancer are now on patient labels.[98] The powerful pharmaceutical lobby fought the FDA on this matter through the courts. But in the end, two Federal appeals courts supported the agency's position, and patient labels have been required since 1977 (for postmenopausal estrogens) and 1978 (for oral contraceptives).

This should be convincing evidence, to women, that exogenous estrogens should be used with grave caution, and avoided whenever possible.

Segaloff and Maxfield[99] suggested the possibility of there being a synergistic carcinogenic action between estrogens and X-radiation, and thereby raised an important clinical question: should an asymptomatic woman who has taken large quantities of hormones—and who is, presumably, at higher risk—be screened by mammography? So far, no one has offered a solution to this new quandary women are facing.

Other, nonsteroidal hormones have also been studied, and insulin[100] and relaxin[101] appear to play some role. Epidemiological data suggest that diabetic women are at a somewhat higher risk; the possible involvement of relaxin may explain the relationship between lower rates of breast cancer in women having early menarche and menopause as well as the enigma (to women) about the importance of having a first child before the age of 18.

In 1976, Kapdi and Wolfe[102] caused a brief scare when they reported finding high-risk duct patterns in the xeromammograms of women taking thyroid medications. However, this subsided when epidemiological data showed it was having hypothyroidism that was the high-risk factor—not the medication used for treating it.[103]

Jick,[104] director of the Boston Collaborative Drug Surveillance Program, raised the question of the use of reserpine for hypertension, because the substance was shown to elevate serum prolactin levels. Since this hormone has long been associated with mammary carcinogenesis, the FDA warned physicians about its potential dangers in a special bulletin.[105] Many physicians are now using substitute hypotensive drugs to lower the blood pressure of possible high-risk patients.

Although certain pituitary hormones seem to play a role in the etiology of some mammary carcinomas, these are of little practical interest to women at this time.

In the area of viral research, Schlom et al.[106] continued their investigations of a possible human mammary tumor virus, but—despite excellent experimental designs—conclusive data have been elusive. They have found that the suspicious "particle" (or virus) may be transmitted not only by milk or by gametes, but also by the placenta and seminal fluid. Again, this research stresses that any virus—when and if it is discovered—will probably not, itself, be the only cause of breast cancer.

At some point, laboratory research into the etiology of breast cancer merges with epidemiological research, and so these joint findings will be discussed together. For example, the role of genetics, as far as humans are concerned, can best be investigated by surveying large populations of breast-cancer patients. Indeed, there is strong epidemiological evidence that the disease does "run in the family."[107-109] Moreover, there are data from Iceland[110] indicating that the paternal genetic heritage is as important as is the maternal. There is also some evidence showing that any history of cancer in either side of a woman's family may increase her risk of developing breast cancer; i.e., the organ where a possible oncogene may begin to grow varies, and a child may not develop the same cancer the parent had.[111]

In 1969, Hakama[112] had reported a curious statistical phenomenon—"Clemmesen's hook"—and suggested that there may actually be two distinct types of breast cancer, pre- and postmenopausal, each having different etiologies and requiring different treatment. By 1980, this hypothesis had gained support from epidemiological statistics.[113] Women whose mothers or sisters developed the disease premenopausally are at higher risk themselves, especially if the disease was bilateral. On the other hand, women whose first-degree relatives were not diagnosed until they were older have lower risks. These risks are further reduced as the relatives' age at the time of diagnosis advances. In other words, if a woman's mother or sister was 65 or more when the disease was discovered, her risk is probably the same (9%) as that of the rest of the general female population in the United States.

Another interesting factor pertaining to family history is that daughters of premenopausal breast-cancer patients—if they develop the disease at all—will do so as much as 5 years earlier than their mothers did.

Identical twins are difficult to find, but there are two pairs in the records of the Breast Cancer Advisory Center. In one family, both sisters developed breast cancer premenopausally: one had bilateral disease, and the second has had one mastectomy. In the second pair, the sister who took diethylstilbestrol (DES) during pregnancy has *not* developed breast cancer, while her twin—who never took the estrogen—developed bilateral disease.[46]

Continuing epidemiological studies support earlier data regarding the importance of the length of a woman's reproductive life and the age when her first child was born. Nulliparity still carries a high-risk label, but it has been established that women who have never had children at all have a lower risk than do those who gave birth to their first child after the age of 30.

Some European scientists question the inference drawn by MacMahon and Cole that breast feeding makes no difference, arguing that women in the United States do not have many children and do not breast-feed them as long as do women living abroad. According to this hypothesis, the protection conferred by breast feeding two or three children for 6 months each is not significant, while nursing five children, each for 3 years or even longer, would inhibit the development of disease.[114]

Are emotions involved in the etiology of breast cancer?

The possible role of emotional factors, particularly of stress, became a popular subject in the lay press in the 1970's.[115] Although most of the published data were based on so-called "soft" scientific approaches (batteries of subjective psychological tests and evaluations[116]), there was some "hard" evidence as well. For example, there are studies associating stress with immune suppression, and the latter has been shown to be linked with the cause of some cancers in animals.[117] The fact that the hypothalamus controls emotions as well as pituitary activity also suggests such a hormonal interaction.[118] Future interdisciplinary efforts in research should clearly be valuable. There is, at this time, at least one such joint project between the NCI and the National Institute of Mental Health. This work involves the possible role that certain emotional characteristics may play in prolonging the lives of malignant-melanoma patients.[119]

Scientists frequently view attempts to measure emotions with skepticism, but a patient sees the absence of such research as a stubborn refusal to try new approaches. Letters to the Breast Cancer Advisory Center have come from many women who developed breast cancer *after* having been prescribed various antidepressants.[46] Although this is "anecdotal evidence," it does suggest a correlation between diagnosed affective illness and subsequent diagnoses of the disease. The possibility that affective illness plays some role in the etiology of breast cancer should not be ignored simply because such research is difficult.

Biological psychiatry now has the expertise and technology to quantify some of the psychobiological serum and urinary markers associated with acute stress, using scientific methods that should satisfy even the most stringent criteria. It was suggested that the Breast Cancer Task Force of the NCI collaborate in doing a prospective study of some of these psychobiological markers in breast-cancer patients. However, the idea was not pursued.[120]

In the meantime, newspapers, magazines, and books are linking all types of emotional problems with breast cancer. Anxious to prevent the disease, women are turning to expensive psychotherapy, biofeedback, transcendental-meditation courses, and other "antistress" regimens, even though they may be of little value.[121]

The role of nutrition in the etiology of breast cancer has also become a popular concern, because knowing the cause should result in a way to prevent it. In 1979, public pressure pursuaded the director of the NCI, Arthuc C. Upton, to give the Senate an "anticancer diet."[122] True, laboratory research has shown that foods do affect breast-cancer development,[123] and epidemiological evidence has supported these findings. It is well known, for example, that Japanese women who adopt the dietary habits of either Hawaii or the mainland United States eventually develop the same high incidence rates as do Caucasians.[124] Studies in Japan have shown a 25% rise of breast-cancer incidence in urban women who have adopted Western diets, e.g., more meat and less seafood.[125] A joint United States–Japan committee has already held several meetings in Seattle to look into the role of diet in the etiology of breast cancer.

Second-generation Jewish women whose parents emigrated to New York from Europe also developed more breast cancer than their mothers did.[126] Phillips[127] has shown that Seventh Day Adventists (who eat no meat or animal fats) have low breast-cancer incidences; Mormons (who eat little of these foods) have a somewhat higher rate, but it is still lower than most women's in the United States.[128]

Recently, milk and milk products, rather than meat and animal fats, have been implicated. There are also epidemiological data to support this finding, since countries in which large quantities of milk, butter, and cheese are eaten usually appear at the top of world-incidence tables and charts.[129]

Laboratory studies have shown that depriving $A \times C$ mice of calories, whatever their source, reduces the rate of mammary carcinoma by as much as two thirds.[130] This animal research has been borne out in humans by follow-up studies of concentration-camp survivors who were starved before and during World War II. Modan[131] reported that the incidence of breast cancer in these Jewish women—usually a high-risk group—is lower than that of other Israeli women, except for those whose ancestries are Mediterranean—Sephardim. This group has one fourth the incidence of others in the country and is the subject of intense investigation by virtually all disciplines involved in breast-cancer research.

For scientists, low-risk populations—Israeli Sephardic, rural Japanese and Finnish, poor black women in the United States—and of high-risk groups—nuns, the British, Irish, Scandinavian, and Dutch, and the Parsi women in India—are sources of valuable data. DeWaard[22] based his theory about total body volume, i.e., height as well as weight, on such subgroups. The knowledge that low-risk women have higher titers of estriol[94] and that their estrogen fractions differ from those of high-risk women[95] is also a result of studying these women.

Parsi women have many times the incidence that other populations in India have.[132] Is this because they are more affluent and have better diets, take estrogens, and go to college, avoiding childbirth until they are older? Or is it because they have been isolated and inbred for centuries?

Heredity?

Do Sephardic Israeli women—usually from north African or Middle East countries—have better genes than their Ashkenazic (northern European and American) sisters do? Or is it their poverty?

Affluence?

In the United States, being black has long been considered as "protective," and yet a study of black women living in Washington, D.C.[113]—a city where the black population earns more per capita than anywhere else in the U.S.—showed the breast-cancer incidence to be the same as that of the city's whites. Does this explain why American Indians and Hispanics have lower incidences? Is affluence the reason urban Japanese women are developing more disease?

Add the odd fact that wet earwax seems to be associated with high risk while dry earwax is a low-risk indicator,[134] and the picture is even more confusing.

But these "indicators" can, at least, be seen and measured. Fraumeni et al.[135] have identified certain parts of the United States where breast-cancer mortality is highest. Almost invariably, "hot spots" on the map designate highly industrialized areas where unseen and unmeasurable pollutants may be affecting the incidence of breast-cancer development. There is little, if anything at all, to be done about studying these at this time.

But epidemiological and laboratory research have recently been enhanced by a change in world politics, and this has resulted in pooling international data and scientific exchanges. Because of obvious differences in geography, economics, and life styles (especially of diet) around the world, such biomedical cooperation should certainly contribute a great deal of knowledge.

But now, women see the etiology and epidemiology of this bizarre disease as a convoluted mystery that will be unraveled only by a medical Sherlock Holmes.

4.3. Detection and Diagnosis

What women need is a "Pap smear" for breast cancer.

Mammography, xeromammography (xerography or xeroradiography), thermography, ultrasonography, radioactive scintigraphy, and other -graphies are expensive, time-consuming gadgets for women who are truly "affluent." So are infrared brassieres and computerized axial tomography (CAT) scanners. Unfortunately, while having money (and all that being affluent involves) appears to raise breast cancer risks,[136] being poor does not make a woman immune. Biological, histological, immunological, and biochemical markers—whether found in blood, urine, aspirated nipple fluid, or the tissue of a benign lesion—may some day result in a safe, cheap, quick, and easy Pap smear. So, to women, the experimental biologists working in these fields are as deeply involved in detection as are radiologists and ultrasonographers.

It is unnecessary to cite the statistics of breast cancer here, but these are constantly being given to women by all the media: one of every 11 women living in the United States today will develop breast cancer at some time in her life, and its incidence is higher in those subgroups identified in Section 4.2. As a result, millions of women live in fear that something is growing in their breasts.

From a patient's point of view, there are four areas for which some-type of marker is needed.

1. For identifying benign lesions that are true precursors of breast cancer, so these women may be properly monitored or conservatively treated or both.
2. For the detection of subclinical primary breast cancer.
3. For identifying certain characteristics of a tumor that could be prognostic and assist women and their surgeons in the choice of adequate primary treatment.
4. For the detection of occult micrometastases so that appropriate anticancer therapy can be administered or changed (for those already receiving adjuvant treatment of some kind) while the tumor burden is minimal.

Except for research related to HANs, little has been published regarding the characteristics of suspicious benign tissue. Since having a history of nonmalignant breast disease is an indicator that a woman is at higher risk of eventually developing cancer, more such research might be extremely valuable.

The little that has been published seems promising. Gullino[137] and Folkman et al.[138] have been studying the degree of angiogenesis of a benign lesion and of the area around it. Haagensen[139] has described certain markers he considers to be important in identifying subgroups of patients who should be carefully monitored for breast cancer. And, of course, Gallager and other pathologists[140] are continuing their studies of hyperplasia and other preneoplastic conditions. Except for these few efforts, there appears to be a dearth of research into this important early-detection area. Yet finding such markers would benefit the hundreds of thousands of women in the world who are terrified that their chronic benign diseases have targeted them for inevitable breast cancer.

Petrakis[33] and his colleague Sartorius seemed to be on the verge of developing a simple Pap test using a special pump to aspirate nipple fluid. This work is still ongoing, but the results have been variable in terms of false-negative diagnoses. While there is still hope for improvement in the future, women must now depend on clinical (too often, inadequate) examination and mammography to find a breast lesion as early as possible.

Thermography—a technique for measuring heat retention of diseased tissue—was evaluated in comparative trials as a part of BCDDPs, discussed elsewhere in *Breast Cancer* and in this chapter. Because it is a noninvasive modality, advocates of its use as a breast-screening method believed that thermography would replace the use of ionizing radiation—especially for younger women. Unfortunately, this hope was not realized: the technique resulted in enough inaccurate results that its use in the BCDDPs was ultimately limited only to those screening centers in which research to perfect it further is being done.[141]

A complicated and lengthy procedure, ultrasonography still appears to be a promising early-detection tool. However, so far, analyzing the sound-pictures is highly subjective, and the technique is far from ready to be used on the community level. Chang[142] first reported his successful use of CAT scanning for finding subclinical breast lesions in 1978. While CAT scanning may prove to be an accurate and reliable modality, it will probably never be practical as a mass-screening device because of its considerable cost.

Thus, mammography of some kind—reproduced on film or on Xerox paper—is at this time the most reliable way to detect subclinical lesions, as a partner to good clinical examination.

The controversy regarding the potential radiation risks of mammography has been discussed elsewhere in *Breast Cancer* and will not be repeated here. However, it must be pointed out that even if mammography were 100% free of radiation risk and 100% accurate, the vast majority of women could still not benefit from it: it is not economically feasible. Four breast X-rays and a clinical examination can cost from $75 to $200. For working women, the cost of losing time from work and of travel to and from a radiologist's office must also be taken into account.

Most third-party carriers—including Medicare—do not pay for screening of any kind, even if women are older than 50. Therefore, the expense of this detection modality makes regular mammographic screening prohibitive for most women in the United States. But even if the cost is not a problem, asymptomatic women younger than 50 cannot have the comfort and security offered by mammography unless they are first-degree family histories. Since premenopausal women frequently have chronic cystic problems, this group has a special need for a noninvasive detection modality, and it is imperative that a safe, easy, less expensive early-detection method be developed.

Wolfe[143] has had promising results in predicting high-risk subgroups of women on the basis of ductal parenchymal patterns, and these are being studied by other investigators (with some controversy and disagreement). However, these prognostic indicators depend on xeroradiography for, at least, a base-line mammogram, and the problems of cost again interfere with its use by the average woman. Moreover, the Bureau of Radiological Health (BRH) has found that equipment using xeroradiography exposes a woman to as much as 4.5 times as much ionizing radiation as film-screen mammography does. Thus, the

NCI recommendations pertaining to women below age 50 would prohibit wide use—regardless of the reliability of Wolfe's data.[144] For example, if a woman's base-line xeroradiogram at age 30 showed her to be at high risk, future screening by any type of mammography would be contraindicated.[145]

To sum up these early-detection modalities from a woman's point of view, none is feasible or practical for use as a routine screening technique. Either their cost, time and inconvenience involved, unreliability, or possible risks of radiation (at this time) rule them all out for use by asymptomatic women. The only method that offers any possibility for mass, routine breast-screening is a marker that is present in the blood or urine or one that can be elicited by a simple and easy test such as Springer's T-antigen.[146]

Herberman[147] has detailed the current "state of the art" in Vol. 2 of this series. For the purpose of this patient-oriented chapter, it is sufficient to enumerate the 10 areas of current research he outlined:

1. Oncofetal antigens
2. Placental markers
3. Breast- or milk-associated antigens
4. Other ectopic hormones
5. Enzymes
6. Normal body constituents
7. Histopathological markers
8. Alteration in immune functions
9. Immune responses to breast-cancer-associated antigens
10. Antigen–antibody complexes

To a patient, it seems as though one of these ten areas of research should have yielded something that is specific to early breast cancer. However, all such marker studies seem to have ended in blind alleys, so far as detecting primary disease is concerned.

Another population of women in urgent need of a marker are those who have had surgery for localized disease and are worrying about having a possible metastasis develop elsewhere in their bodies. Some women had negative axillary nodes but are nonetheless aware that there may be micrometastases in other organs; some had positive axillary nodes but were not given adjuvant therapy for a variety of reasons; others are receiving adjuvant therapy of some kind. But none has any way of knowing whether or not she is truly free of disease: only the presence or absence of a metastatic lesion on scan or X-ray is a marker for these women.

The problem is acute for those whose adjuvant regimens cause severe toxicity, and postmenopausal women are especially affected. The reason for this is simply that there have been numerous articles in the lay media reporting the possible ineffectiveness of cytotoxic agents in this age group. Therefore, older women have the added stress of thinking, "Is it worth it?" even though data keep appearing showing improved results with larger doses.

If cancer never reappears, the adjuvant therapy is considered successful. But if it does recur, only then do women know that the agents did not stop the progress of the disease in their cases. Hundreds of letters and telephone calls to the Breast Cancer Advisory Center indicate that this uncertainty has become a high-priority problem, and finding some kind of a marker for micrometastases is now imperative.

There are some efforts being made in this important area. Since 1976, Dao and Ip[148] have been using serum sialyltransferase levels to monitor the progress of women being treated for advanced metastatic disease, as well as of symptom-free women receiving adjuvant chemotherapy and patients whose only treatment was primary surgery. Preliminary results[149] show a correlation between elevations and evidence of disease or its progression. Decreases in the enzyme level are associated with decreases of tumor burden; women whose serum sialyltransferase levels remain within normal limits have continued to be disease-free. Kessel et al.[150] Lipton et al.[151] and Walkes[152] are working along the same lines.

Marker research is usually funded by grants, and it is virtually impossible to know what studies are being done, and by whom, until their results are published. Unlike contractors, whose tasks are clearly specified in an RFP (Request For Proposal), grantees are allowed to deviate from their original goals. For this reason, this author is unaware of other related research, and any oversight is inadvertent.

A marker of some kind is also needed to stage the tumor itself to try to find an indicator that may predict whether or not the woman is a high risk of developing a recurrence. There seems to be general agreement that the presence or absence of disease in the axilla is a primitive and unreliable method for determining whether additional treatment of some kind is needed,[56] and most anticancer agents are too toxic to give every woman who has surgery for local disease. Yet, at this time, all adjuvant therapy is being administered on the basis of a woman's nodal status. Rich,[153] Nealon,[154] Black,[155] Friedell et al.[156] and many other investigators are working on this problem.

Why have markers been such stepchildren of breast-cancer research? One reason has been the absence of reliable technology for measuring trace quantities of any substance. Radioimmunoassay is a relatively new technique, and little marker research could be done before it was developed. Moreover, until the advent of breast self-examination, mammography, and other early-detection modalities, women rarely presented until they had advanced disease. Therefore, prognoses were inevitably bleak, and there was no need for sophisticated studies of the tumor to attempt to either minimize primary treatment or predict future outcome. Without effective anticancer agents, a marker that might pick up an occult metastasis was useless: nothing could be done even if one were discovered. Progress has changed this grim picture, and it is now urgent that markers be found to help in every stage of the disease.

According to Hilf,[157] another reason for the lack of success has been that there is not enough recognition of markers' importance. This view is shared by others, among them Schwartz,[158] McIntire,[159] Wells,[160] Acevedo,[161] and Tormey.[162] As a rule, an absence of recognition also means a lack of cooperation from scientists working in other areas. For example, pathologists might establish a "bank" of hyperplastic or other suspicious benign lesions, a bank where specimens could be sent for future research. Radiologists could, perhaps, freeze blood and urine specimens of asymptomatic women. Since about 7% of them will eventually develop breast cancer, any marker they may have in common could be important. Although technology may not yet have reached the stage where such specimens are useful, the time to begin collecting material is now; waiting for the appropriate apparatus to be invented could mean additional years of delay.

The Health Insurance Plan (HIP) in New York had the foresight to anticipate this possibility as early as the 1960's, when blood specimens were routinely taken from women screened at the Guttman Institute. Unfortunately, most of these specimens thawed during New York's electrical blackout of 1965, but the collection has since been resumed (with an emergency generator available should there be another power failure). Those samples that were not ruined are in frozen storage at the Mayo Clinic.

Strax[163] and Hayward are currently collaborating in a trans-Atlantic study of the blood that was (and is being) collected at Guttman, since the blackout occurred. As screenees develop breast cancer, their specimens are sent to Hayward in London, where any shared biological, biochemical, or immunological markers are studied.

Since breast cancer is a multifactorial disease, it seems, from a patient's point of view, that this type of cooperative, interdisciplinary research is invaluable. Obtaining the data depends on all scientists, working in different research areas, to combine forces to achieve a common goal. Nowhere is this need more evident than in the search for elusive markers.

The discovery of the importance of estrogen receptors is an excellent example of the progress that has been made in differentiating among the many types of breast cancer. In the past, a tumor was diagnosed only for its histological information: benign or malignant. Now, it has been proven that cancer cells have other characteristics as well—estrogen (and other steroids) receptors. These studies were originally basic research into finding the reasons for the presence or absence of these proteins. Yet, within a few short years, their role in terms of choosing appropriate therapy and for predicting more favorable outcomes has shown that nuclear typing and nuclear grading of a tumor are not enough. It is now essential that the tumor be studied for its estrogen dependency as well. If the same effort is applied to other characteristics of a breast-cancer cell, similar therapeutic and prognostic indicators will certainly be found.

No discussion of breast-cancer detection can be complete without some mention of the BCDDPs—the Breast Cancer Detection Demonstration Projects—sponsored jointly by the NCI and the American Cancer Society (ACS). They have received so much attention in both the lay and the professional media that it is unnecessary to go into detail here. Their most publicized problem—the so-called "66 benigns"—were banner-headlined in most of the country's newspapers and magazines. Yet, the final outcome of the re-re-review of these women's pathologies was given little publicity. By the time the Working Group—chaired by Oliver Beahrs—published its final report in mid-1979,[164] the "mammography controversy" was long since over as far as the public was concerned.

During the intervening two years—September 1977 to September 1979—enough had been published and broadcast to do both harm and good. Women who should have continued to be screened (i.e., those older than 50 or over 40 with strong family histories) were flocking away from mammography in the same large numbers that flocked to be X-rayed after the Betty Ford–Happy Rockefeller mastectomies in 1974. The Breast Cancer Advisory Center has records of several dozens of women who should have continued to be screened but who refused any further exposures to X-ray. This, plus the expenditure of tens of millions of dollars, is the harm. But, as stated earlier, there was also some good, and lessons were learned from the outcome of this well-intentioned program.

The first is the recognition that no definitive treatment should be performed on the basis of a brief frozen-section pathological study in the case of lesions smaller than 1 cm.[165] If several pathologists had been given the time to study the 66 "questionable"[164] slides, women would not be afraid they would have unnecessary mastectomies as a result of participating in a screening program.

Second, large-scale programs to detect any cancer should have some kind of built-in mechanism for following their participants. This last factor was inherent in the HIP study, on which the BCDDPs were based. Because HIP is a prepaid health insurance plan, it was able to have easy access to information about patients' subsequent treatment. The BCDDPs, on the other hand, were free-standing detection centers, and results from mammograms were sent to the women's private physicians. Thus, there was no straightforward procedure to inform either the ACS or the NCI about the women's treatment afterward. Although physicians and hospitals usually cooperated and submitted information, doing so was voluntary; some did not.

This was one of the major causes of the confusion surrounding the September 1977 National Institutes of Health (NIH) Consensus Development Conference convened to discuss the BCDDPs.

The third benefit from the projects has already been discussed in detail: the great need for a method to ascertain nodal invasion, disseminated disease, and multicentricity. It is unreasonable to expect a woman to try to find a microscopic, subclinical breast lump, only to be treated with the same radical surgery used when lesions are the size of walnuts or lemons.

However, by far the most important outcome of the BCDDPs was a quick and sharp reduction of the excessive doses of ionizing radiation being emitted by the X-ray equipment.[166] As a result of the massive publicity, the BRH and the NCI began a cooperative program to inspect and monitor the mammography apparatus in the BCDDPs. Moreover, all X-ray units used throughout the country to examine women's breasts (about 6000) are being upgraded to meet the criteria of the bureau's Mammography Quality Assurance Program. The American College of Radiology is cooperating with the BRH to reduce radiation levels, consistent with good quality. Industry has also helped by manufacturing low-dose film that can produce excellent images of the contents of a breast without requiring large quantities of radiation.

Thus, despite some of the deleterious aftereffects of the BCDDPs, women have benefited from them: radiation levels have been reduced, and there is more quality control over mammography.

However, it is still too expensive to be routine, and even those women who can afford it have the omnipresent dread that early detection may result in an unnecessary mastectomy. All of the well-intentioned scientists involved in breast-cancer detection, diagnosis, and treatment must realize that this fear is uppermost in the minds of most women.

4.4. Primary Treatment

Surgical procedures used to treat primary breast cancer have been discussed throughout this chapter. They are: the supraradical mastectomy with *en bloc* removal of the chest wall; the Halsted (classic or standard) radical mastectomy; the modified radical mastectomy (now renamed the total mastectomy with axillary dissection); the total mastectomy (formerly known as the simple) with only a sampling of the axillary nodes; quadrantectomy (also known as "wide excision" or "wedge excision") with or without postoperative axillary dissection or biopsy, with or without irradiation of the remainder of the breast; segmental resection (also called "local excision," "lumpectomy," or "tylectomy") with a complete axillary dissection or only an axillary sampling and with or without irradiation of the preserved breast. When irradiation is substituted for a mastectomy, the X-ray therapy may or may not involve the use of radioactive implants in the area where the lesion had been embedded.[167]

This diverse list of current primary therapies may remind many readers of the varied menu of a New York delicatessen. The only item missing from this menu is a needle biopsy followed by primary radiotherapy, a procedure often done in other parts of the world. And if a woman in the United States searches diligently enough, she could undoubtedly find someone here who offers this treatment.

The confusion is exacerbated by information from a 1979 report issued by the American College of Surgeons.[168] It tells that a survey of United States hospitals, for 1977, found that there were 14 different types of breast cancer among 23,777 cases treated in that year. These were: "*in situ* [lobular or ductal], Paget's, lobular infiltrating, ductal infiltrating, papillary, scirrhous, medullary, colloid, comedocarcinoma, inflammatory, adenocarcinoma [NOS], carcinoma [NOS], other, [and] > 1 histologic type." While these cases were varied by the American College of Surgeons according to cell type, there were other variables not mentioned in the report. For example, the size of the tumor, its location, and the age of the woman are factors that might have influenced a surgeon's treatment choice.

Women who are aware of this multitude of permutations and combinations of treatment options need a fourth-generation computer to help program their therapy. The most difficult thing for women is knowing that the bottom line of all of them is identical: differences in the survival rates of the women treated by this wide variety of procedures are not statistically significant, no matter what was done. The yardstick against which all primary breast-cancer surgery has been measured for almost a century—the Halsted radical mastectomy—is not fail-safe. Overall, a woman who develops breast cancer has a 50–50 chance of being alive in 10 years. By now, everyone who reads newspapers, magazines, and books, listens to the radio, or watches television knows this grim statistic.

Yet, despite the multitude of variables and procedures, 91.8% of the

24,136 cases of breast cancer included in the survey were treated by some type of mastectomy. The Halsted radical was done 48.4% of the time, regardless of any other factors involved.[168] It seems as though breast cancer is thought of as a ruptured appendix: a mechanical problem that can be corrected in the same way in every body.

The American College of Surgeons' report surveyed treatments used in 1977, and extrapolating from this base, it was clear that the popularity of the Halsted was decreasing. Only about 25,000 of these procedures would have been done in 1978, and it was assumed there would be even fewer in 1979.[168]

Because of this surgical change of habit, the NIH convened an international Consensus Development Conference on June 5, 1979, to discuss "The Primary Treatment of Breast Cancer: Management of Local Disease." Members of the panel were: John Moxley, Chairman, John R. Durant, Bernard Fisher, Samuel Hellman, Rose Kushner, Bernard Pierquin, Jerome Urban, Umberto Veronesi, Joseph C. Allegra, Jane Henney, and Franco Muggia. This author, a nonphysician, abstained from any participation in the debate regarding the type of surgery to be done.

At the end of a day of often heated discussion, it was the consensus of the panel that "a procedure which preserves the pectoral muscles, i.e., a total mastectomy with axillary dissection, provides equivalent benefit to women who have Stage I and selected Stage II breast cancer. Therefore, total mastectomy with axillary dissection should be recognized as the current treatment standard."

Urban opposed a phrase of the recommendation describing axillary dissection as a staging procedure rather than a therapeutic one: Fisher questioned inclusion of the term "selected Stage II." The final recommendation was therefore a compromise—agreed to by the entire panel. At the urging of this author, the Consensus Development panel also recommended that "a two-step procedure should be done in most cases, i.e., a diagnostic biopsy should be studied by permanent histologic sections before definitive therapeutic alternatives are discussed with the patient." The panel agreed that since there is no medical or surgical reason for following the diagnostic biopsy immediately by any definitive treatment, such a recommendation should be adopted for women who desire a delay between the two procedures.

Veronesi supported the recommendation for its psychological benefits to women; Pierquin and Hellman agreed, because a woman would not have an opportunity to investigate alternatives if her breast were removed immediately; Fisher argued that separating the diagnosis from treatment is logical, because of the need to stage the extent of a patient's disease before any definitive therapy is considered; Urban felt a waiting period to be unnecessary for his own patients, but agreed that it might be beneficial to those women whose surgeons do not take as much time to explain available options as he does.

Fisher's comments regarding the need for premastectomy staging are especially important to women, because the American College of Surgeons' report showed that 56.74% of patients with Stage IV disease, women having distant metastases at the time of primary treatment, had some kind of mastectomy, nonetheless. Such a high rate of mastectomies in cases where metastatic disease is already present at the time of diagnosis must have been due to the fact that the surgeries were done on the basis of the frozen-section pathology report. Thus, separating the diagnostic biopsy from any further treatment will serve two purposes:

1. Women whose breast cancers have already spread beyond the axillary lymph nodes will no longer be subjected to any surgery, except whatever may be needed to remove as much tumor as possible from the gland.
2. Women will have time to investigate ongoing clinical trials comparing lesser surgeries on a controlled basis, if they could choose to do so.

Endorsement of these clinical trials was the third recommendation of the Consensus Development panel. Specifically, the panel supported "further clinical investigation into the roles of segmental mastectomy and primary radiotherapy . . . in regard to answering the question about the effectiveness of lesser surgical procedures in women with Stage I and Stage II carcinoma of the breast. These ongoing clinical trials, because of their exciting preliminary results, warrant support both from patients and physicians so that the continuing search for the optimal patient treatment can progress to the point of maximal patient survival and minimal patient morbidity."

Thus, women in the United States have entered an era where they must know more about breast cancer to make informed, intelligent decisions. This means that the waiting period recommended by the NIH will be useless unless physicians and surgeons agree to give patients information about the relative benefits and risks of all available alternatives. They must also be willing to refer women to clinical trials, if they should want to look into these.

Although the panel made no recommendations about preoperative staging examinations, these are vitally important to women. However, their value appears to be a source of disagreement, even among breast-cancer experts. Urban[169] and Robbins[170] believe that such presurgical examinations are unnecessary unless the patient has complaints or symptoms. On the other hand, Dao,[171], Leis[172], Schwartz,[173] and others do skeletal surveys routinely before any definitive treatment is done. If the patient chooses to have the diagnostic biopsy and mastectomy (if necessary) combined in a single procedure, staging examinations are done beforehand. [172]

Johnston and Jones [174] have reported the detection of occult skeletal metastases by scintigraphy as early as 22 months before these became symptomatic or could be visualized on conventional X-rays. As mentioned elsewhere, the yield of micrometastases in distant organs—by scintigraphy or other techniques—is still too small to justify their use as a basis for the surgical management of breast cancer. However, even if these relatively crude modalities had permitted only 10% of 1979's breast-cancer patients to be diagnosed if they had metastatic disease, staging would have prevented the unnecessary removal of almost 11,000 breasts in that year.

A technological miracle that seemed to be a boon—reconstructive mammoplasty—may yet prove to be women's bane. Breast reconstruction is undoubtedly a physical and psychological marvel for those women whose breasts have already been or must be removed because of invasive cancer. However, the procedure is not—and should not be considered to be—an "alternative treatment" for chronic fibrocystic disease, hyperplasia, or other types of benign disorders, or for being at high risk. This author has frequently heard the statement, "If there's any doubt that it might turn into cancer, just do a mastectomy; she can always get reconstruction afterward." Lynch [175] made front-page news by recommending bilateral, prophylactic mastectomies for high-risk young women. In addition, it has become common for women calling the Breast Cancer Advisory Center to report that they were advised to have a "prophylactic" mastectomy with a subsequent implant, when they were treated for carcinoma in the contralateral breast, "just in case...." [46]

Of course, an absent organ or limb cannot develop cancer, so it is not difficult for surgeons to convince these women that a prophylactic mastectomy is the "safest" course of action. While there are instances when some type of prophylactic plastic surgery is indicated, wholesale advocacy of such procedures appears to have become routine postmastectomy advice on the part of many surgeons. [176]

Reconstructive mammoplasty should be discussed in the later section devoted to the psychological aspects of breast cancer (Section 4.6), because the procedure is of greatest value in this area. However, it is being mentioned here because there is a recent trend toward combining preparations for future plastic surgery with the initial treatment. There are even some surgeons who are performing both simultaneously, in a single procedure. Most breast-cancer experts, however, believe nothing should be done until the incision is well healed and the skin is pliable.[177] Others prefer waiting 18–24 months, because they fear that an implant may hide a recurrence.[178] Many cancer surgeons are now consulting with plastic surgeons to plan the primary treatment with future reconstruction in mind. For example, whenever possible, the areola and nipple are "banked" so they can be grafted onto the breast mound later.[179]

Manufacturers of implants are constantly improving them, and plastic surgeons are perfecting new techniques. If a woman is willing to undergo several procedures (and can afford them), it is even possible to graft skin and muscle from other parts of her body to correct the chest-wall and axillary defects caused by extensive radical surgery.

Those women whose areolas and nipples were lost may have new ones created from labial skin; a bit of ear cartilage is used to elevate the center to resemble an erect nipple.[180] There are surgical complications in many cases, complications that involve the implant's rejection, sloughing, and hardening (known as "contracture"), as well as the ordinary problems of infection and hematoma.[181] Moreover, Snyderman[182] has described the new "breast" as being far from "a cosmetic triumph."

Nonetheless, for women who have had mastectomies, reconstructive mammoplasty offers cosmetic benefits that external prostheses cannot match. From a medical point of view, Urban[183] and others believe that the availability of this procedure will induce women to seek professional help more quickly after finding a symptom of breast cancer. This, they feel, will decrease the number of women who die of the disease.

The costs of reconstructive mammoplasty vary upward from $1000 (excluding hospitalization) and depend on the degree of surgery required as well as on the general fee schedule for a particular geographic area. Although most third-party carriers still consider the procedure to be cosmetic, the American Society of Plastic and Reconstructive Surgeons has been effective in obtaining coverage in many states.[184]

4.5. Adjuvant Therapy and Metastatic Disease

The decade began with the recognition that some type of adjuvant chemotherapy, given immediately after primary surgical treatment, had been effective in delaying recurrences in premenopausal women with positive axillary nodes. As described earlier, the NSABP's decision to conduct controlled clinical trials using some kind of adjuvant chemotherapy was based on the success of cytotoxic drugs in causing regressions and remissions in women with advanced disease. These first drugs were triethylenethiophosphoramide and 5-flourouracil, administered within the first week after the mastectomy was performed.[61] Since the histories of early trials using various agents are well chronicled in *Breast Cancer: Advances in Research and Treatment,* Vol. 1, by Fisher and Wolmark,[185] and Carbone and Tormey,[186] it would be redundant to repeat them.

However, writing as a counselor to women undergoing postoperative therapy, as either an adjuvant (for those symptom-free) or for metastatic disease, presents an opportunity to discuss the subject from the patient's point of view. All the information in the following pages is based on letters and telephone calls from women who have had questions, worries, and anxieties about their treatment (or, often, nontreatment). These are not random samples, and they may not be representative of the majority of breast-cancer patients. However, this information does give an insight into the kinds of problems some women are experiencing, and for many readers, it may offer an opportunity to better understand their patients' attitudes. Many clinicians may be surprised; many may think these problems do not actually exist—at least, not as far as their own patients are concerned.

On the other hand, for many readers, this information will reinforce something they already know: breast-cancer patients today are pioneers who are assisting scientists in the exploration of uncharted territory. And many realize full well what vital roles they are playing in medical history. But while they know it must be done and that they must be on the forefront, it is not easy. They need emotional support that is, unfortunately, often not available from their physicians or surgeons. Thus, these pages are being written with the hope that knowing a little about patients' problems will enable both clinicians and researchers to help them cope with their fears and uncertainties.

Perhaps the most frightening aspect of receiving any therapy now is that of being a "guinea pig."

So far as primary treatment is concerned, this pertains mainly to the use of ionizing radiation. Any mention of damaged nuclear plants or disasters involving radiation is, as a rule, accompanied by information explaining the potential dangers of the invisible rays. Women get scared. But since patients receiving irradiation instead of surgery usually elected to do so with full knowledge that its long-range effects are still unknown, they are inhibited from discussing their fears. These women are reluctant to talk to the radiotherapist, because they feel that doing so would seem to be an accusation that he or she might be harming them. Unlike women who have mastectomies, they usually do not confide even in members of their families or close friends, because primary radiotherapy is considered unorthodox.

In particular, they do not have the comfort available from groups such as Reach to Recovery, because most of their members had mastectomies and have a tendency to resent anyone who decided to "play Russian roulette" by having less surgery. They also have the added burden of being unsure that radiation therapy may be as effective, in terms of survival, as surgery. For these women, the only sources of emotional support and strength are the radiation therapist, members of his or her staff, and other patients receiving the same primary treatment. It is a difficult time psychologically as well as physically.

As far as postoperative adjuvant treatment is concerned, not all clinicians are convinced that such prophylactic treatment should be used, because they believe an axillary dissection is, in itself, curative. Physicians holding this philosophy give nothing to their patients, and these women worry about *not* getting pills or shots when everyone they know with positive nodes is getting something.

There is also disagreement about postmenopausal women vis-à-vis cytotoxic agents, since so many data showed these drugs to be ineffective for delaying recurrences in this age group. Again, there is worry about getting nothing.

The permutations and combinations of drugs used for adjuvant chemotherapy and their schedules are—like primary treatments—mind-boggling. If one counts endocrine manipulation for estrogen-receptor-positive, positive-node patients—oophorectomy, adrenalectomy, hypophysectomy, tamoxifen, aminoglutethimide, alone or in combination—a patient's confusion and bewilderment can be appreciated.

Patients who meet in a physician's waiting room are probably treated in the same way, a treatment based on the same philosophy. But waiting rooms are not the only places where women meet. There is also the checkout line at the supermarket; there are carpools, PTA meetings, church socials, dinner parties, and political coffees. Breast-cancer patients do not live in a vacuum where only their personal clinicians' views prevail.

What happens when women compare notes?

Ms. Green, who had ten positive nodes, is getting CMF, but now she wonders if she would not be better off with FAC. Ms. Brown was randomized into a protocol based on estrogen-receptor status, and she has learned that others in the same trial are getting tamoxifen; she is not. Ms. Smith, who had one positive node, wonders why Ms. Jones—who also had a single node—is so lucky. Her doctor believes in no drugs at all. So Ms. Jones is not vomiting, nor is her mouth always sore. Most important, she is not wearing a wig. Although physicians consider alopecia to be a minor side effect of cytotoxic drugs, to women it is often the most critical: not only were they forced to lose a breast, but they must also lose the crowing glory of femininity—their hair.

Women wonder why there are so many differences of opinion, and they worry. Of course, the reason is simply that no one yet knows what is the best treatment for all women. Only when all the clinical trials and protocols have accumulated 5 or 10 years' worth of recurrence and survival data will computers have enough information to tell scientists which agent, which combination, and which schedule have the best results for each category of patients. In the meantime, everyone receiving therapy today is a pioneer for future generations.

But even pioneers worry. Every breast-cancer article in a tabloid newspaper is read voraciously, and when a "breakthrough" is announced in a more prestigious publication, many women want to abandon whatever regimen they are on to take advantage of the miraculous new "cure." Often, preliminary results of investigational substances are given as "background" information to medical writers, and these are reported in the lay press. Substances such as thymidine, interferons, and vaccines, new or more potent drugs combinations, immune therapies, or experimental treatment by unusual apparatus—hyperthermia, lasers, or fiber optics—have appeared, often prematurely, in highly reputable newspapers and magazines. In their confusion and bewilderment, patients already receiving therapy interpret promising results, in small samples of patients over short periods of time, as proven treatment—if only they could be admitted to the center where these are available.

Again, the discussion must return to the urgent need for a simple, inexpensive, and reliable marker that could tell women and their physicians if their therapy is being effective. Most of all, a marker could predict which one of every four node-negative women is harboring a micrometastasis somewhere in her body.

Women who have not had breast cancer hope scientists will develop a vaccine to prevent the disease altogether; their second-best research choice is some way to detect a subclinical primary lesion so that a mastectomy of any kind will not be necessary. Of course, women who have already been treated for primary disease—those receiving nothing, adjuvant therapy, or treatment for mestastases—are beyond this point: these patients fervently hope a cure for breast cancer is just around the corner.

But their second-best hope is control. They will settle for a medication, such as insulin, that must be taken forever if only it will control the fatal spread of the disease and save their lives.

4.6. Psychosocial Aspects of Breast Cancer

The psychosocial aspects of breast cancer are usually thought of entirely as the psychosocial aspects of *mastectomy*—the variety of psychiatric problems in adjusting to life with one breast or none, loss of femininity, sexuality and body image, and other concerns. To scientists, clinicians, and women with advanced disease, controversies regarding primary surgery seem relatively unimportant, because the disease is so lethal. Patients with metastatic disease worry about living; fears women may have about the type of initial surgery are only a tip of the iceberg that simply ceases to matter.

However, none of these areas received much attention in the past, because quantity of life, *not* its quality, was everyone's main concern. Only when women began to live longer *with* the disease was "coping with cancer" finally recognized to be the serious problem that it is.[187]

The "psychosocial aspects of breast cancer" is therefore a broad term that actually covers far more than merely the problems of breast loss. In 1974, this author evolved a "psychological clinical staging" outline of the presurgical anxieties, based on questionnaires and interviews of 130 women who had had mastectomies.[188] During the succeeding two years, letters and telephone calls to the Breast Cancer Advisory Center made it clear that the five phases identified at that time were insufficient. A revised chronology of psychological–clinical staging was adopted.[189] These included:

1. Anxieties of asymptomatic women (often beginning in their teens) about developing the disease.
2. Anxieties of symptomatic women watching and waiting or anticipating diagnosis and treatment.
3. Anxieties associated with primary treatment, adjuvant therapy, and disseminated disease.
4. Anxieties associated with treatment failure and impending death.

Within each phase, there are subcategories of other problems, each peculiar to that phase.[190] The use of the term "psychosocial aspects of breast cancer," rather than of only mastectomy, has permitted health professionals to adapt these clinical stages as devices for crisis-intervention techniques.[191,192]

However, there is one psychological symptom that pervades all the phases—denial: refusal to know or to accept the truth. Denial can be a healthy defense mechanism that protects a dying patient from losing her equilibrium entirely, or it can be a dangerous, suicidal barrier to finding and treating an early, potentially curable breast cancer. Indeed, denial is an overwhelming component of the psychosocial milieu that surrounds breast phase and stage of this disease, and it may very well be a major contributor to its high mortality rate.

4.6.1. Asymptomatic Women

What is known about the presurgical fears women have about breast cancer?

In 1973, the ACS commissioned the Gallup organization to interview 1007 women over the age of 18. The report, "Women's Attitudes Regarding Breast Cancer,"[193] showed that 56% considered this disease to be the most serious medical problem facing them. Of these, 77% had known someone personally who had the disease; 41% knew three or more breast-cancer patients. When the women in the survey were asked to estimate the number of women out of every 1000 who developed breast cancer, 56% guessed the number to be 100 or more—greater than the actual incidence rate in the United States. More than one third of those polled (38%) believed that half or more of all lumps in a breast are cancerous. Moreover, 39% believed that a diagnosis of breast cancer meant certain and imminent death, while only 26% believed that "a great deal" of progress had been made against the disease.

This Gallup poll showed that the level of anxiety, fear, and panic felt by healthy women over the age of 18 is formidable.

In response to these data, the ACS, the NCI, the American Medical Association, and other related organizations began planning programs to battle the undue fear and pessimism by disseminating more accurate and optimistic information about incidence and survival. Along with such "fear-reduction" programs, women were encouraged to practice regular breast self-examination (BSE), and subsequently, the BCDDPs were inaugurated nationally. The goal of all the publicity was to save lives by bringing breast cancer "out of the closet" for diagnosis while the disease was still "early" and therefore curable.*

The assumption that women will do anything to detect an early symptom is based on two premises that are not necessarily valid: (1) that all women fear the loss of their lives more than they fear the loss of their breasts ard (2) that women believe earlier diagnosis and treatment can eradicate the disease from their bodies with absolute certainty.

In view of the wide publicity given to unchanged mortality rates of the previous three decades—even with early detection—these proved to be less than accurate assumptions. Much was written about the natural biology of breast cancer after 1974, and many women learned that small

---

*In November, 1980, the National Cancer Institute announced the results of another poll by the Opinion Research Corporation. The emphasis on breast self-examination would now be accompanied by more direct instructions by medical professionals.

lesions are not necessarily "early" lesions. And, of course, there has been a great deal of publicity about the worldwide controversies regarding the efficacy of extensive surgery as opposed to conservative procedures. This has added to women's confusion. Finally, the outcome of the BCDDPs (the "66 questionable cases") convinced millions of women that finding a suspicious spot too early could mean the unnecessary loss of a breast.

Advocates of early detection should understand that what they are urging women to do is a classic example of an operant-conditioning paradigm.[194] Essentially, women are being told to perform a complex, expensive, and perhaps risky series of behaviors to find something they do not want to find. Then, if they do as they were instructed and discover a lump or thickening, their "reward" will usually be the amputation of their breasts. Small wonder that fewer than 25% of all women practice regular self-examination.[193] Behavioral scientists are not surprised at this finding, because it is well established that threats of punishment (aversive control) rarely maintain desirable behaviors, while consequences that are positively reinforcing will result in the expected performance.[195] Yet early-detection programs are predicated on the notion that normal women will actively seek out a symptom that will cause them to be punished.

If any kind of mastectomy were a guaranteed cure, this notion might make sense. However, at this time, no one can give such a guarantee: all that can be done now to reduce the severity of the consequences of early detection is to tell women that if a cancer is found early and their axillary lymph nodes are negative, they have a 75% chance of being alive in 5 or 10 years.

Of course, there have been advances that have changed the consequences of early detection, but they are so recent that their effects cannot yet be evaluated. For example, the June 5, 1979, Consensus Development Conference recommended that a total mastectomy with an axillary dissection (formerly known as the modified radical mastectomy) become the treatment of choice for most cancers of the breast, rather than the disfiguring Halsted or standard radical mastectomy. In addition, the conference recommended that there be an interval between the diagnostic biopsy and definitive treatment.

By issuing this single statement, the consensus panel eliminated one of women's major fears concerning breast cancer: the dread of being wheeled into an operating room without knowing, in advance, whether they will awaken with one breast or with two.

Finally, progress in reconstructive mammoplasty has given new hope to women who have already had mastectomies in the past and to those who will face the loss of their breasts in the future.

Most of these changes affect either symptomatic women or those who have already been diagnosed. But what of the millions of women represented by the 1007 interviewees of the Gallup poll, the totally asymptomatic women?

As mentioned earlier, the recommendation that the diagnostic biopsy be separated from definitive treatment—if followed by all surgeons—would eliminate the most terrifying of these fears: not knowing before the biopsy what the outcome will be. However, there are others.

For asymptomatic woman over the age of 35, the constant threat of breast cancer is, in itself, an emotional problem that can cause either obsessive fear or strong denial. Of the two, denial is far more serious, because these women usually refuse to learn anything about the disease, do not examine themselves, and will not see their physicians for clinical examinations.

This situation is apparent in the 1973 ACS poll. Of the women interviewed, only 77% had ever heard of BSE, and only 3 of 10 had ever practiced it, even occasionally. Although ignorance was a factor in some cases, many women who knew about the need for monthly BSE cited "fear and anxiety" as their reason for not doing so. Almost half (46%) felt that such monthly self-checks "would make them worry unnecessarily." There were more subtle indications of denial, such as "Neglect," "Should have but haven't taken the time," and "Don't feel like I have a need for it."[193] Obviously, this preclinical phase of denial, despite intense fear of developing breast cancer as its cause, can cost women their lives.

4.6.2. Symptomatic Women

Denial is also the reason women delay in consulting a physician. This problem is so common that it has even been given a name by psychiatrists and psychologists—"lag time."[196]

The ACS and the NCI estimate that 110,000 new cases of breast cancer were diagnosed in 1981—a statistic that means that about 535,000 women in the United States had some type of breast-cancer symptom (since eight of every ten lesions are found to be benign). Using these United States data as a base, more than a half million women in this country went through the anguish and anxiety of worrying about having breast cancer in that year, even though only 20% were found to have the disease. According to interviews of hundreds of women anticipating breast biopsies in the United States,[46] the presurgical phases of emotional trauma are far more difficult than are the postsurgical problems, excepting those of patients having advanced disease.

Such strong fear reactions almost invariably result in strong denial and avoidance behaviors.

But once this denial is overcome and an appointment is finally requested and obtained, women must wait for the day and scheduled time. For men and women alike, any medical examination is traumatic whenever a symptom of the "Big C" is concerned, and the waiting is often exquisitely painful. Finally, when the examination is over and the clinician does find something suspicious, even more waiting is involved, where breast cancer is concerned: another menstrual cycle or two, attempts at aspiration, endless lines at the radiologist's office for mammograms, days, perhaps weeks, of waiting for a slot in a hospital's operating-room schedule for a biopsy. Before even facing the swinging doors of the operating room, however, there are interminable admissions procedures, preoperative laboratory tests and X-rays, and the emotional gamut associated with any hospital stay—children, babysitters, and becoming accustomed to a strange and fearful environment.

For those women without adequate insurance coverage, the economics of a simple diagnostic biopsy may add to the existing trauma. Including the expense of the operating and recovery rooms, anesthesia, medication, work-ups, and so on, this preliminary surgery may cost $500 or more for an overnight stay. The surgeon's fee, of course, would be additional.

Women who have a symptom of breast cancer must endure all these traumas. Their anxiety is acute, and clinicians can be of great help in lessening the problem by being available for support personally, or by having a sympathetic nurse or other health professional available to answer questions. The clinician may also be invaluable by eliminating as much waiting time and delay as possible.

If the biopsy's result is "benign," a woman's immediate agony is over. For those diagnosed to have cancer, however, there are still presurgical X-rays, scans, and laboratory tests to be done. Fears about these (in particular, any test involving radiation or radioactivity) can be assuaged if the women are told what is to be done to them and the reasons for doing it.

For premenopausal women who are frequently cystic, there are additional emotional problems. Normal cyclical changes frequently mimic breast cancer, and younger women must often endure months of watching and waiting before they are even considered candidates for surgical biopsies.

Too frequently, denial steps into the watch-and-wait ordeal, and women simply decide to do nothing more. They do not read about the disease in newspapers, magazines, or books; they push it to the backs of their minds. "If I know too much, I'll get it" is a common attitude.

Or "If it's going to hit me, there's nothing I can do about it" is another, potentially lethal, point of view. These are the women who—if they finally visit a clinician—usually have numerous positive axillary nodes or may even already have symptoms of metastatic disease.

Yet, as important as denial is to early detection of breast cancer, little work has been done to study its prevalence or what to do about its existence.

4.6.3. Treatment

Several of the early traumas involved with the treatment of primary breast cancer have already been mentioned: presurgical X-rays, radioactive scans of all types, and laboratory tests. Knowing that these are essential to stage the extent of disease and to determine whether or not the patient is a candidate for any kind of breast surgery adds fear to the miscellaneous procedures. On the other hand, there is some benefit— the intervals between tests and examinations permit women to accept their diagnoses and even to look forward to surgery, because they are operable.

Clinicians managing women during this phase can help by emphasizing the importance of negative (i.e., hopeful) findings. Oncological social workers and other allied health professionals point out the importance of having time to mourn a loss and to bid farewell to a prized part of the body[197] as a therapeutic measure. For women who grew up in an era of patients' and consumer rights, the knowledge that they are actively involved in all the procedures related to the decision-making is an additional benefit of the waiting period between a diagnostic biopsy and definitive treatment.[198]

Many women will use this time to obtain additional opinions regarding the histology, learn of alternative treatments, and consult with plastic surgeons about future reconstructive procedures. By the time definitive treatment is imminent, they are prepared emotionally for whatever is to happen. At this time, their major fear will concern the presence of positive axillary nodes.

Of course, the foregoing list of emotional benefits vs. emotional traumas can result only if the clinician is aware of and sensitive to the frequently unspoken fears of his patient. If a woman is not permitted to know what is being done to her and why the procedures are important, the clinician is more likely to encounter intense rage, hostility, and depression after the surgery is completed. Being "duped" is a common complaint.[46]

Three decades ago, women who lost breasts to cancer were isolated in a world of their own. Artificial breasts to help them look and feel normal had to be fabricated with rags, absorbent cotton, and bird seed. Lead sinkers used by fishermen were often recommended to "weight" the lumpy pouch for large-breasted women, so they would not suffer from spinal pain caused by the change of balance.

All that is history. There are now about 100 commercial prostheses available, and some are even tinted to match women's clothing. "Coping with cancer" has become a popular area for health professionals: there are now oncological social workers, nurses, psychotherapists, thanatologists, and other specialists in related disciplines who are interested in helping cancer patients deal with all aspects of their disease.

As a result, the clinician need not be alone in helping a breast-cancer patient cope with the side effects of adjuvant radiation therapy, chemotherapy, or endocrine manipulation. However, the increasing number of women receiving such treatment—especially adjuvant chemotherapy—has created a new area of denial: many women resent or even refuse these continuing treatments, because they are constant reminders of having the disease.

Unlike women receiving therapy for metastases, those on adjuvant regimens are free of symptoms of their diseases, and the injections (and their sequelae) are not thought of as being immediately helpful. No pain disappears; no tumor shrinks. The only cause of their being bald, nauseous, or tired is the medication—not the disease it is treating. It is easy for these women to abandon adjuvant treatment at the first hint in lay or professional media that it may prove to be useless.

The fears of those women who have received primary treatment and who must wait 5 or 10 years to know whether they are out of danger of a recurrence of disease have been discussed elsewhere. Until 1974, they had other problems as well.

Reach to Recovery was the first program to help with day-to-day practical solutions: exercises to rehabilitate the affected arm, lists of the few stores where breast prostheses and special clothing were sold. It also offered a clublike atmosphere where mastectomy patients can meet and feel free of the stigma of having lost one or both breasts. It must be remembered that breast cancer was—and in some areas still is—considered a secret social disease.

Until the autumn of 1974, when Betty Ford and Happy Rockefeller courageously told the world of their mastectomies, the only well-known women who had told of their surgeries publicly were Shirley Temple Black and Marvella Bayh. When the Ford–Rockefeller mastectomies made the disease mentionable, more "personalities" admitted their surgeries as well—but only a few.

The sudden open attitude about breast cancer brought unknown breast-cancer problems into the public eye. For example, the fact that job and credit discrimination exist against women who have had the disease was given publicity.[199] It is difficult for them to obtain insurance for ten years, and moreover, their husbands are "second-hand" victims, because their medical insurance policies usually cover the women as well. Thus, they cannot change jobs unless the same third-party carrier is also used elsewhere. When adjuvant therapy became routine, its cost added to the need for the husband to stay in the same job. Such economic problems are as "psychosocial" as are psychiatric problems.

The psychosocial aspects of advanced disease and impending death, so far as breast-cancer patients are concerned, do not differ from those of other terminally ill people. For this reason, readers should refer to the work of recognized authories—Kubler-Ross,[200] Stoddard,[201] Saunders,[202] Krant,[203] and others—who have contributed to a better understanding of this final phase.

However, one aspect that affects scientist, clinician, and patient alike is the politics of cancer. Most readers will immediately think in terms of grants, contracts, peer-review, and Congressional appropriations at the mention of the word "politics." This is not the case: the true politics of cancer will not be found in a study group or even in the office of the director of the NCI.

The politics of cancer rest in the Congress and in the ubiquitous bureaus, offices, agencies, and boards that regulate life in the United States. Excessive radiation dosage is the domain of the Bureau of Radiological Health, the Environmental Protection Agency, the Nuclear Regulatory Commission, and perhaps even more. The FDA's Bureau of Drugs is responsible for approving or disapproving medications; the Social Security Administration deals with covering the costs of all medical care involving women over the age of 65.

Third-party coverage for prostheses—external as well as internal—is not universal: the sovereign states regulate what a Blue Cross–Blue Shield plan will be required to pay. Widows and divorcees, as well as unmarried women, frequently have inadequate insurance coverage for the considerable costs of primary surgery. If any type of adjuvant therapy is indicated, this will probably not be included. Yet, because of other income or property, these women are not eligible for government aid unless they are older than 65.

The FDA has been accused of delaying the approval of useful, proven medications. However, many third-party carriers still do not reimburse patients for the antiestrogen tamoxifen, even though it has been declassified as "experimental" since the end of 1977. And, as mentioned earlier in this chapter, breast-screening by mammography is not covered, unless the clinician indicates the presence of a possible cancer symptom.

In May 1979, Massachusetts enacted legislation requiring physicians to inform women about all the alternatives involved in breast-cancer treatment, and their benefits and risks. This state also requires X-ray technologists to be certified and has ordered third-party carriers to cover reconstructive mammoplasty as "rehabilitative surgery" rather than as a cosmetic procedure. In all cases, political pressure was used to legislate medical care. These are but a few examples of the "real politics" of cancer—the kinds of politics that are involved in petitions, lobbying, and elections. It is unlikely that many scientists have ever considered these issues when they think of "the politics of cancer."

As emphasized at the beginning of this chapter—its "prologue"—patients view breast cancer differently from scientists and clinicians. This glimpse of some of the political issues may be surprising to those who have little time and few opportunities to learn about the day-to-day practical problems that patients encounter as they cope with this disease.

On the other hand, patients have little patience with what appears to be the snail pace of medical progress in finding a way to prevent, control, or cure cancer. Reading the kinds of problems discussed in *Breast Cancer: Advances in Research and Treatment* is of great help in enabling a patient to understand the enigmatic puzzle of cancer. Unfortunately, the language of science is too difficult for popular consumption, and the public can learn only via "translations" in the mass media. Cross-pollination, however, is essential. Just as it is beneficial to put a patient into a scientist's seat—even for a few hours—it is hoped that the reverse will also be true.

5. References

1. S. S. DeVesa and D. T. Silverman, Cancer incidence and mortality trends in the United States: 1935–74, *J. Natl. Cancer Inst.* **60,** 545–571 (1978).
2. Conquest of Cancer Act: Report No. 92-247, Calendar 239, Hearings Re: S1828, 92nd Congress, June 28 (1971).
3. M. B. Shimkin, As memory serves—an informal history of the National Cancer Institute, 1937–57, *J. Natl. Cancer Inst.* **59,** 559–600 (1977).
4. N. I. Berlin, Introduction: The breast cancer task force, in: *Report to the Profession: Breast Cancer,* pp. 1–10, Breast Cancer Task Force, National Cancer Institute, Bethesda, Maryland (1974).
5. G. Crile, Jr., *What Women Should Know About the Breast Cancer Controversy,* Macmillan, New York (1973).
6. J. Gershon-Cohen, S. M. Berger, and H. S. Klickstein, Roentgenography of breast cancer moderating concept of "biologic predeterminism," *Cancer* **16,** 961 (1963).
7. B. Fisher and N. H. Slack, Number of lymph nodes examined and the prognosis of breast cancer, *Surg. Gynecol. Obstet.* **129,** 709 (1969).
8. B. Fisher, N. H. Slack, and I. D. J. Bross (and cooperating investigators), Cancer of the breast: Size of neoplasm and prognosis, *Cancer* **24,** 1071–1080 (1969).

9. B. Fisher and E. R. Fisher, Role of the lympathic system in the dissemination of tumor, in: *Lymph and the Lymphatic System* (H. S. Myerson, ed.), pp. 324–347, Charles C. Thomas, New York (1968).
10. B. Fisher and E. R. Fisher, Transmigration of lymph nodes by tumor cells, *Science* **152**, 1397–1398 (1966).
11. M. F. Burnet, Immunological factors in the process of carcinogenesis, *Br. Med. Bull.* **20**, 154–158 (1964).
12. G. T. Beatson, On the treatment of operable cases of carcinoma of the mamma: Suggestions for a new method of treatment with illustrative cases, *Lancet* **2**, 104, 162 (1896).
13. E. V. Jensen and H. I. Jacobson, Basic guide to the mechanism of estrogen action, *Recent Prog. Horm. Res.* **18**, 387 (1962).
14. D. H. Moore, J. Charney, B. Kramarsky, E. Y. Lasfarques, N. H. Sarker, M. J. Brennan, J. H. Burrows, S. M. Sirsat, J. C. Paymaster, and A. B. Vaidya, Search for a human breast cancer virus, *Nature (London)* **229**, 611 (1971).
15. J. J. Bittner, Possible method of transmission of susceptibility to breast cancer in mice, *Am. J. Cancer* **39**, 104 (1940).
16. R. L. Carter, Immunological control of metastatic growth, in: *Host Defense in Breast Cancer: New Aspects of Breast Cancer* (B. A. Stoll, ed.), pp. 6–35, Year Book Medical Publishers, Chicago (1974).
17. C. K. Wanebo, K. G. Johnson, K. Satok, and T. W. Thorslund, Breast cancer after exposure to the atomic bombings of Hiroshima and Nagasaki, *N. Engl. J. Med.* **279**, 667–671 (1968).
17a. S. Jablon and H. Kato, Mortality among A-bomb survivors, 1950–1970, *JNIH-ABCC Life Span Study*, Report 6, Technical Report 10–71 (1971).
18. A. N. Papaioannou, *The Etiology of Human Breast Cancer*, pp. 170–77, Springer-Verlag, New York, Heidelberg, and Berlin (1974).
19. *Competitive Problems in the Drug Industry*, United States Senate, Vols. 1–3, parts 15–17, Hearings of the Subcommittee on Monopoly of the Select Committee of Small Business, 91st Congress: Oral Contraceptives, Feb. 24, 25; March 3, .4 (1970).
20. F. G. Arthes, P. E. Sartwell, and E. F. Lewison, The pill, estrogens and the breast: Epidemiological aspects, *Cancer* **28**, 1391 (1971).
21. B. MacMahon, P. Cole, and J. Brown, Etiology of human breast cancer: A review, *J. Natl. Cancer Inst.* **50**, 21 (1973).
22. F. W. deWaard, Breast cancer incidence and nutritional status with particular reference to body weight and height, *Cancer Res.* **35**, 3351–3356 (1975).
23. L. Venet, P. Strax, W. Venet, and S. Shapiro, Adequacies and inadequacies of breast examinations in mass screening, *Cancer* **28**, 1777–1785 (1971).
24. A. Salomon, Beiträge zur Pathologie und Klinik der Mammakarzinome, *Arch. Klin. Chir.* **101**, 573–668 (1913).
25. J. Gershon-Cohen and A. Streckler, Roentgenologic examination of the normal breast: Its evaluation in demonstrating early neoplastic changes, *Am. J. Roentgenol.* **40**, 199–201 (1938).
26. R. L. Egan, Experience with mammography in a tumor institution, *Radiology* **75**, 894–900 (1960).
27. P. Strax, L. Venet, S. Shapiro, and N. Gross, Mammography and clinical examination in mass screening for cancer of the breast, *Cancer* **20**, 2189 (1967).
28. P. Strax, L. Venet, and S. Shapiro, Mass screening in mammary cancer, *Cancer* **23**, 875–878 (1969).
29. A. I. Holleb, Testimony before the Health Subcommittee of the House of Representatives, June 1977.

30. K. Lloyd-Williams, F. Lloyd-Williams, and R. S. Handley, Infrared thermometry in the diagnosis of breast disease, *Lancet* **2,** 1378 (1961).
31. W. Pomerance, The breast cancer demonstration projects, in: *Report to the Profession: Breast Cancer,* pp. 119–126, Breast Cancer Task Force, Bethesda, Maryland (1974).
32. L. Breslow, A brief chronology and commentary on the controversy regarding mammography for women under 50, in: *UCLA Bulletin,* pp. 3–4, November 12 (1976).
33. N. L. Petrakis, Breast fluid as a diagnostic tool, in: *Report to the Profession: Breast Cancer,* pp. 133–146, Breast Cancer Task Force, Bethesda, Maryland (1974).
34. G. Baum, Development of ultrasound mammography, in: *Report to the Profession: Breast Cancer,* pp. 127–132, Breast Cancer Task Force, Bethesda, Maryland (1974).
35. T. M. Chu and T. Nemoto, Evaluation of carcinoembryonic antigen in human mammary carcinoma, *J. Natl. Cancer Inst.* **51,** 1119–1122 (1973).
36. D. C. Tormey, T. P. Walkes, D. Ahmann, C. W. Gehrke, R. W. Zumwatt, J. Snyder, and H. Hansen, Biological markers in breast carcinoma. I. Incidence of abnormalities of CEA, HCG, three polyamines, and three minor nucleosides, *Cancer* **35,** 1095–1100 (1975).
37. R. C. Coombes, T. J. Powles, J. C. Gazet, H. T. Ford, J. P. Sloane, D. J. R. Laurence, and A. M. Neville, Biochemical markers in human breast cancer, *Lancet* **1,** 132–134 (1977).
38. M. M. Black, S. R. Opler, and F. M. Speer, Survival in breast cancer in relation to the structure of the primary tumor and the regional lymph nodes, *Surg. Gynecol. Obstet.* **100,** 1580 (1971).
39. H. J. G. Bloom and J. R. Field, Impact of tumor grade and host resistance on survival of women with breast cancer, *Cancer* **28,** 1580 (1971).
40. S. J. Cutler, M. M. Black, and I. S. Goldenberg, Prognostic factors in the female breast: An investigation of some interrelations, *Cancer* **16,** 1589 (1963).
41. C. S. B. Galasko, Screening for the potentially curable patient, in: *Breast Cancer Management: Early and Late* (B. A. Stoll, ed.), pp. 15–23, Year Book Medical Publishers, Chicago (1977).
42. C. Rhoads, Report on a cooperative study of nitrogen mustard (HN_2) therapy of neoplastic disease, *Trans. Assoc. Am. Physicians* **60,** 110–117 (1948).
43. C. D. Haagensen, *Diseases of the Breast,* W. B. Saunders, Philadelphia (1971).
44. J. A. Urban, Therapy of primary cancer, *Calif. Med.* **112,** 10–13 (1970).
45. H. P. Leis, Jr., Selective breast cancer surgery: Is there a place for less than radical mastectomy?, *Int. Surg.* **61,** 76 (1976).
46. The Breast Cancer Advisory Center (1975–79).
47. R. M. Gregorio and B. Fisher, The pathology of invasive breast cancer: A syllabus derived from findings of the National Surgical Adjuvant Breast Project (Protocol No. 4), *Cancer* **36,** 1 (1975).
48. D. H. Patey and W. H. Dyson, The prognosis of carcinoma of the breast in relation to the type of operation performed, *Br. J. Cancer* **2,** 7–13 (1948).
49. J. A. Urban and M. A. Marjani, Significance of internal mammary lymph nodes metastases, *Am. J. Roentgenol.* **1,** 130–136 (1971).
50. U. Veronesi and L. Zingo, Extended mastectomy for cancer of the breast, *Cancer* **20,** 677–680 (1967).
51–52. B. Fisher, Surgery of primary breast cancer, in: *Breast Cancer: Advances in Research and Treatment,* Vol. 1, *Current Approaches to Therapy* (W. L. McGuire, ed.), pp. 22–27, Plenum Press, New York (1977).
53. R. G. Ravdin, B. Fisher, E. G. Lewison, N. H. Slack, and T. L. Dao, A clinical trial concerning the worth of prophylactic oophorectomy in the treatment of breast cancer, *Surg. Gynecol. Obstet.* **131,** 1055–1064 (1970).

54. E. C. Easson, Post-operative radiotherapy in breast cancer, in: *Symposium on Prognostic Factors in Breast Cancer*, pp. 118–127, Livingstone, Edinburgh (1968).
55. B. Fisher and N. H. Slack, Number of lymph nodes examined and the prognosis of breast cancer, *Surg. Gynecol. Obstet.* **131**, 79 (1970).
56. DeMoss, E., Personal communication (November 1979).
57. D. Schottenfeld, A. G. Nash, G. F. Robbins, and E. J. Beathe, Jr., Ten-year results of the treatment of primary operable breast carcinoma: A summary of 304 patients evaluated by the TMN system, *Cancer* **38**, 1001 (1976).
58. U. Kim, Factors influencing metastasis of breast cancer, in: *Breast Cancer: Advances in Research and Treatment*, Vol. 3, *Current Topics* (W. L. McGuire, ed.), pp. 21–24, Plenum Press, New York (1979).
59. National Cancer Institute Research Report, *Drugs vs. Cancer*, pp. 1–4, DHEW No. (NIH) 75-786 (1974).
60. P. P. Carbone, The role of chemotherapy in treatment for breast cancer, in: *Cancer Chemotherapy—Fundamental Concepts and Recent Advances*, pp. 311–322, Year Book Medical Publishers, Chicago (1975).
61. B. Fisher, R. G. Ravdin, R. K. Ausman, N. H. Slack, and R. J. Noer (and cooperating investigators), Surgical adjuvant chemotherapy in cancer of the breast: Results of a decade of cooperative investigation, *Ann. Surg.* **168**, 337–356 (1968).
62. National Cancer Institute Report, *End Results in Cancer: Report No. 4*, pp. 99–103, DHEW No. (NIH) 73-272 (1972).
63. B. Fisher, Primary therapy of breast cancer, in: *Report to the Profession: Breast Cancer*, pp. 157–170, Breast Cancer Task Force, National Cancer Institute, Bethesda, Maryland (1974).
64. I. MacDonald, The breast, in: *Management of the Patient with Cancer* (T. F. Nealon, ed.), pp. 435–469, W. B. Saunders, Philadelphia (1965).
65. A. A. Fracchia, J. H. Farrow, and A. J. dePalo, Castration for primary inoperable or recurrent breast carcinoma, *Surg. Gynecol. Obstet.* **128**, 1226 (1969).
66. O. H. Pearson, at: National Institutes of Health Consensus Development Conference on "Steroid Receptors in Breast Cancer," Bethesda, Maryland, June 27–29 (1979).
67. T. Lasser, Reaching the patient with breast cancer, in: *The Breast* (H. S. Gallager, ed.), pp. 326–332, C. V. Mosby, St. Louis (1978).
68. N. Bard and A. N. Sutherland, Psychological impact of cancer and its treatment. IV. Adaptation to radical mastectomy, *Cancer* **8**, 655–672 (1955).
69. V. Barckley, Enough time for good nursing, *Nurs. Outlook* **12**, 44–48 (1964).
70. J. Holland, Psychosocial aspects of breast cancer, Presentation before the XIIth International Cancer Congress, Buenos Aires (1978).
71. M. J. Asken, Psychoemotional aspects of mastectomy: A review of recent literature, *Am. J. Psychiatry* **132**, 56–59 (1975).
72. T. D. Cronin, J. Upton, and J. M. McDonough, Reconstruction of the breast after mastectomy, *Plast. Reconstr. Surg.* **59**, 1–14, (1977).
73. H. D. Harrel, To lose a breast, *Am. J. Nurs.* **72**, 676–677 (1972).
74. R. Kushner, After surgery: Psychological, in: *Breast Cancer: A Personal History & an Investigative Report*, pp. 230–258, Harcourt Brace Jovanovich, New York (1975).
75. H. S. Gallager and R. V. P. Hutter, Pathology and pathogenesis of breast cancer, in: *The Breast* (H. S. Gallager, ed.), pp. 49–50, C. V. Mosby, St. Louis (1978).
76. K. B. DeOme, Formal discussion of multiple factors in mouse mammary tumorigenesis, *Cancer Res.* **25**, 1348–1351 (1965).
77. H. P. Leis, Jr., Breast cancer: Patients at risk, presented before the Third International Symposium on Detection and Prevention of Cancer, New York (1977).

78. P. Cole, Epidemiology of breast cancer: An overview, *Report to the Profession: Breast Cancer*, pp. 11–20, Breast Cancer Task Force, Bethesda, Maryland (1974).

79. H. S. Gallager and J. P. Martin, A study of mammary carcinoma by correlated mammography and subserial whole organ sectioning: Early observations, *Cancer* **23**, 855–873 (1969).

80. E. R. Fisher, Pathology of breast cancer, in: *Breast Cancer: Advances in Research and Treatment*, Vol. 1, *Current Approaches to Therapy* (W. L. McGuire, ed.), pp. 92–97, Plenum Press, New York (1977).

81. H. M. Jensen, J. R. Rice, and S. R. Wellings, Preneoplastic lesions in the human breast, *Science* **191**, 295–297 (1976).

82. M. Baum, The curability of breast cancer, in: *Breast Cancer Management: Early and Late* (B. A. Stoll, ed.), pp. 3–13, Year Book Medical Publishers, Chicago (1977).

83. J. F. Egan, C. B. Sayler, and M. J. Goodman, A technique for localizing occult breast lesions, *Cancer* **26**, 32 (1976).

84. D. E. Bauermeister and M. H. Hall, Specimen radiography: A mandatory adjunct to mammography, *Am. J. Clin. Pathol.* **16**, 789–798 (1973).

85. *Cancer Facts & Figures*, American Cancer Society (1979).

86. R. Costlow, Report to the Advisory Board of the NCI Division of Cancer Control & Rehabilitation (October 1978).

87. B. Fisher, Surgery of primary breast cancer, in: *Breast Cancer: Advances in Research and Treatment*, Vol. 1, (W. L. McGuire, ed.), pp. 22–24, Plenum Press, New York (1977).

88. A. C. Upton, Testimony before the Subcommittee on Health, House of Representatives (June 1978).

89. A. C. Upton, L. Breslow, and L. Thomas, Final reports of NCI *ad hoc* working groups on mammography screening for breast cancer and a summary report of their joint findings and recommendations, DHEW No. (NIH) 77–1400, 1–3 (March 1977).

90. E. J. Plata, T. Aoki, D. D. Robertson, E. W. Chu, and B. I. Gerwin, An established cultured cell line (HBT-39) from human breast carcinoma, *J. Natl. Cancer Inst.* **50**, 849–862 (1973).

91. A. Lacassagne, Apparition de cancer de la mamelle chez la souris male, sourise des injections de folliculine, *C. R. Acad. Sci.* **195**, 630–632 (1932).

92. A. Segaloff, Hormones and mammary carcinogenesis, in: *Breast Cancer: Advances in Research and Treatment*, Vol. 2, *Experimental Biology* (W. L. McGuire, ed.), pp. 1–9, Plenum Press, New York (1978).

93. T. L. Dao, Personal communication (1978).

94. H. M. Lemon, Oestriol and prevention of breast cancer, *Lancet* **1**, 546 (1973).

95. M. Kirschner, Relation of endocrine functions to epidemiological characteristics in breast cancer, in: *Report to the Profession: Breast Cancer*, pp. 35–44, Breast Cancer Task Force, Bethesda, Maryland (1974).

96. R. W. Turkington, Multiple hormonal interactions: The mammary gland, in: *Biochemical Actions of Hormones* (G. Litwack, ed.), pp. 55–77, Academic Press, New York (1972).

97. M. E. Lippman, Personal communication (1978).

98. *Physicians' Desk Reference*, 33rd ed., references to hormones: estrogens and progestogen and estrogen combinations, pp. 219–220, Medical Economics, Oradell, N.J. (1979).

99. A. Segaloff and W. S. Maxfield, The synergism between radiation and estrogen in the production of mammary cancer in the rat, *Cancer Res.* **31**, 166–168 (1971).

100. N. D. Cohen and R. Hilf, Influence of insulin on growth and metabolism of 7,12-dimethylbenz(a)anthracene induced mammary tumors, *Cancer Res.* **34**, 3245–3252 (1974).

101. F. Schiotzhe and J. K. McDonald, Relaxin: A disulfide homolog of insulin, *Science* **197**, 914–915 (1977).
102. C. C. Kapdi and J. N. Wolfe, Breast cancer: Relationship to thyroid supplements for hypothyroidism, *J. Am. Med. Assoc.* **236**, 1124–1127 (1976).
103. C. A. Gorman, D. V. Becker, and F. S. Greenspan, Breast cancer and thyroid therapy: Statement by the American Thyroid Association, *J. Am. Med. Assoc.* **237**, 1459 (1977).
104. H. Jick, The Boston collaborative drug surveillance program (1974): Reserpine and breast cancer, *Lancet* **2**, 669 (1974).
105. A. Schmidt, Reserpine reported to increase incidence of breast cancer, FDA Drug Bulletin, September (1974).
106. J. Schlom, D. Colcher, W. Drohan, D. Kufe, and Y. Teramoto, Viruses and mammary carcinoma, in: *Breast Cancer: Advances in Research and Treatment*, Vol. 2, *Experimental Biology* (W. L. McGuire, ed.), pp. 23–46, Plenum Press, New York (1978).
107. D. E. Anderson, Genetic study of breast cancer: Identification of a high risk group, *Cancer* **34**, 1090–1097 (1974).
108. H. T. Lynch, J. Lynch, and P. Lynch, Breast cancer genetics and cancer control: Tumor association, *Arch. Surg.* **110**, 1227–1229 (1975).
109. F. P. Li and J. F. Fraumeni, Jr., Familial breast cancer, soft-tissue sarcomas, and other neoplasms: A familiar syndrome? *Ann. Intern. Med.* **71**, 747–751 (1969).
110. N. Day, Progress report of the International Agency for Research in Cancer to the Breast Cancer Task Force: Breast Cancer in Iceland (January 1978).
111. J. J. Mulvihill, Genetic repertory of human neoplasia, in: *Genetics of Human Cancer* (J. J. Mulvihill, R. W. Miller, and J. F. Fraumeni, Jr., eds.), pp. 137–143, Raven Press, New York (1977).
112. M. Hakama, The peculiar age specific incidence curve for cancer of the breast—Clemmesen's hook, *Acta Pathol. Microbiol. Scand.* **75**, 370–374 (1969).
113. D. E. Anderson, Familial and genetic predisposition, in: *Risk Factors in Breast Cancer* (B. A. Stoll, ed.), pp. 1–24, Year Book Medical Publishers, Chicago (1976).
114. D. B. Thomas and A. M. Lilienfeld, Geographic, reproductive and sociobiological factors, in: *Risk Factors in Breast Cancer* (B. A. Stoll, ed.), pp. 35–39, Year Book Medical Publishers, Chicago (1976).
115. L. LeShan, *You Can Fight For Your Life: Emotional Factors in the Causation of Cancer*, M. Evans, New York (1977).
116. C. Holden, Cancer and the mind: How are they connected?, *Science* **200**, 1363–1369 (1978).
117. M. Stein, R. C. Schiavi, and M. Camerino, Influence of brain and behavior on the immune system, *Science* **191**, 437–440 (1976).
118. V. M. Dilman, Changes in hypothalamic sensitivity in aging and cancer, in: *Mammary Cancer and Neuroendocrine Therapy* (B. A. Stoll, ed.), pp. 197–228, Butterworths, London (1974).
119. N. Rogentine and W. E. Bunney, Jr., Unpublished information.
120. Breast Cancer Task Force: Detection and Diagnosis Committee, May 4 (1979).
121. J. C. Simonton and S. Simonton, Belief systems and management of the emotional aspects of malignancy, *J. Transpersonal Psychol.* **7**, 29–47 (1975).
122. A. C. Upton, Testimony before the Nutrition Subcommittee of the United States Senate, 96th Congress, October 2 (1979).
123. A. B. Miller, Role of nutrition in the etiology of breast cancer, *Cancer* **39**, 2704–2708 (1977).
124. W. Haenszel and M. Kurihara, Studies of Japanese migrants. I. Mortality from cancer and other diseases among Japanese in the United States, *J. Natl. Cancer Inst.* **40**, 43 (1968).

125. T. Hirayama, Socio-economic factors in breast cancer incidence, U.S.-Japan Cooperative Cancer Research Program, Tokyo (May 1976).
126. H. Seidman, Survey of first- and second-generation Jewish women in New York City for the American Cancer Society (1949-51).
127. R. Phillips, Personal communication (1976).
128. J. E. Enstrom, Cancer and total mortality among active Mormons, *Cancer* **42**, 1943-1951 (1978).
129. Cancer Around the World, 1972-1973, in: *Cancer Facts & Figures*, p. 15, American Cancer Society (1979).
130. H. Silverstone and A. Tannenbaum, The effect of the proportion of dietary fat on the rate of formation of mammary carcinoma in mice, *Cancer Res.* **10**, 448 (1950).
131. B. Modan, A dietary study of breast cancer: Progress report to the NCI Breast Cancer Task Force (1978).
132. D. J. Jussawalla, V. A. Deshpande, W. Haenzel, and M. V. Natekar, Differences observed in the site incidence of breast cancer between the Parsi community and the total population of greater Bombay: A critical appaisal, *Br. J. Cancer* **24**, 56 (1970).
133. S. J. Cutler, Newspaper interview: *Washington Star*, February 19 (1979).
134. N. Petrakis, Cerumen genetics and human breast cancer, *Science* **173**, 347 (1971).
135. J. F. Fraumeni, Jr., T. J. Mason, F. W. McKay, R. N. Hoover, and W. Blot, *Atlas of Cancer Mortality for U.S. Counties: 1950-1969*, DHEW Publication No. (NIH) 75-780 (1975).
136. L. A. Brinton, R. R. Williams, R. N. Hoover, S. L. Stegens, M. Feinleib, and J. F. Fraumeni, Jr., Breast cancer risk factors among screening program participants, *J. Natl. Cancer Inst.* **62**, 37-44 (1979).
137. P. Gullino, Angiogenesis and oncogenesis, *J. Natl. Cancer Inst.* **61**, 639-643 (1978).
138. J. Folkman, E. Merler, C. Abernathy, and G. Williams, Isolation of a tumor factor responsible for angiogenesis, *J. Exp. Med.* **133**, 275-288 (1971).
139. C. D. Haagensen, *Diseases of the Breast*, 2nd ed., pp. 155-176, W. B. Saunders, Philadelphia (1971).
140. D. Medina, Preneoplasia in breast cancer, in: *Breast Cancer: Advances in Research and Treatment*, Vol. 2, *Experimental Biology* (W. L. McGuire, ed.), pp. 47-102, Plenum Press, New York (1978).
141. G. D. Dodd and A. Zermeno, Thermography, in: *The Breast* (H. S. Gallager, ed.), pp. 135-140, C. V. Mosby, St. Louis (1978).
142. C. H. Chang, Presentation before the annual meeting of the American College of Radiology, San Francisco, March (1978).
143. J. N. Wolfe, Breast patterns as an index of risk for developing breast cancer, *Am. J. Roentgenol.* **126**, 1130-1139 (1976).
144. P. F. Butler, Current status: Bureau of Radiological Health's Breast Exposure: Nationwide Trends (BENT) program, October 11 (1979).
145. National Cancer Institute, *Mammography: Risks vs. Benefits*, (November 1977).
146. G. F. Springer, Presentation before the annual meeting of the American Chemical Society, Anaheim, and telephone interview by author (November 1978).
147. R. Herberman, Biological markers in breast cancer, in: *Breast Cancer: Advances in Research and Treatment*, Vol. 2, *Experimental Biology* (W. L. McGuire, ed.), p. 217, Plenum Press, New York (1978).
148. T. L. Dao and C. Ip, Alterations in serum glycosyltransferases and 5'-nucleotidase in breast cancer patients, *Cancer Res.* **38**, 723-728 (1978).
149. T. L. Dao, C. Ip, and J. Patel, Serum sialytransferase as a reliable biomarker in breast cancer, *J. Natl. Cancer Inst.* **65**, 3, 529-534 (1980).

150. D. Kessel, T. H. Chou, and M. Henderson, Determinants of fucosyl-transferase level in plasma of the cancer patient, *Proc. Am. Assoc. Cancer Res.* **17**, 16 (1976).
151. A. Lipton, H. A. Harvey, S. Delong, J. Allegra, D. White, M. Allegra, and E. A. Davidson, Gyycoproteins and human cancer. I. Circulating levels in cancer serum, Abstract presented at the 14th annual meeting of the American Society of Clinical Oncology, Washington, D.C. (April 1978).
152. P. Waalkes, The Johns Hopkins Oncology Center, Telephone interview (October 1978).
153. M. Rich, Michigan Cancer Foundation, Telephone interview (October 1978).
154. T. F. Nealon, Discussion at NIH Consensus Development Conference, *The Treatment of Primary Breast Cancer: Management of Local Disease*, June 5 (1978).
155. M. M. Black, Prognostic factors, in: *The Breast* (H. S. Gallager, ed.), pp. 297–319, C. V. Mosby, St. Louis (1978).
156. G. H. Friedell, I. S. Goldenberg, I. J. Masnyk, C. A. McMahan, R. G. Ravdin, J. B. Roberts, A. Segaloff, and F. Welsch, Identification of breast cancer patients with high risk of early recurrence after radical mastectomy. I. Description of study, *J. Natl. Cancer Inst.* **53**, 603–607 (1974).
157–160. R. Hilf, M. Schwartz, K. R. McIntire, and S. A. Wells, Panel discussion on tissue, biological, immunological and simultaneous markers in the diagnosis and monitoring of breast cancer before the semi-annual meeting of the National Surgical Adjuvant Breast Project, Chicago, November 1–2, (1979).
161. H. F. Acevedo, William H. Singer Memorial Research Institute, Telephone interview (May 1978).
162. D. C. Tormey, Personal communication (1976).
163. P. Strax, Guttman Institute, Personal communication (1978).
164. O. H. Beahrs, S. Shapiro, C. Smart, and R. W. McDivitt, Supplemental and concluding report of the working group to review the National Cancer Institute–American Cancer Society Breast Cancer Detection Demonstration Projects, *J. Natl. Cancer Inst.* **62**, 3, 663–672 (1979).
165. National Cancer Institute, Recommendations of the Consensus Development Conference, The Treatment of Primary Breast Cancer: Management of Local Disease, June 5 (1979).
166. T. Judd and R. F. Brown, An evaluation of mammography as a single screening procedure, DHEW Publication No. (FDA) 72-8033, BRH/DMRE 72-6 (1972).
167. J. Vana, R. Bedwani, and G. P. Murphy, Short term patient care evaluation study for carcinoma of the female breast, American College of Surgeons, Commission on Cancer (Preliminary Report), October 12 (1978).
168. J. Vana, R. Bedwani, T. Nemoto, and G. P. Murphy, Long-term patient care evaluation study for carcinoma of the female breast, American College of Surgeons, Commission on Cancer (Final Report), February 21 (1979).
169. J. A. Urban, Preoperative survey, in: *The Breast* (H. S. Gallager, ed.), pp. 147–154, C. V. Mosby, St. Louis (1978).
170. G. F. Robbins, Staging and end-result reporting for patients with breast carcinoma, in: *The Breast* (H. S. Gallager, ed.), pp. 181–191, C. B. Mosby, St. Louis, (1978).
171. T. L. Dao, Personal communication (1974).
172. H. P. Leis, Jr., Presentation before the Gynecological Society for the Study of Breast Disease, April 22–24 (1977).
173. F. G. Schwartz, Jefferson Medical College, Personal communication (1979).
174. G. S. Johnston and A. E. Jones (eds.), *Breast Cancer Diagnosis*, Plenum Press, New York (1977).

175. Auerbach, S., "Pre-center removal of organs urged," newspaper interview, *The Washington Post*, December 4 (1975).
176. G. P. Rosemond, "Breasts are not 'precancerous lesions'," Interview (May 1, 1976, issue Ob. Gyn. News) at American College of Radiology annual conference on breast cancer (1976).
177. R. K. Snyderman, Reconstruction of the breast after mastectomy?, *Ca* **27**, 360–362 (1977).
178. B. Fisher and T. L. Dao, Personal communications (1979).
179. T. M. Biggs, J. Upton, and T. D. Cronin, Reconstruction after mastectomy: How general surgeons can help, *Mod. Med.* May 15 (1978).
180. B. Brent and J. Bostwick, Nipple–areola reconstruction with auricular tissues, *Plast. Reconstr. Surg.* **60**, 353–361 (1977).
181. T. D. Cronin, J. Upton, and J. M. McDonough, Reconstruction of the breast after mastectomy, *Plast. Reconstr. Surg.* **59**, 1–14 (1977).
182. R. K. Snyderman, Reconstruction of the breast, in: *The Breast* (H. S. Gallager, ed.), p. 334, C. V. Mosby, St. Louis (1978).
183. J. A. Urban, Panel discussion at: NIH Consensus Development Conference on The Primary Treatment of Breast Cancer: Management of Local Disease, Bethesda, Maryland June 5 (1979).
184. R. K. Snyderman, Television interview, "Not for Women Only" (January 1977).
185. B. Fisher and N. Wolmark, Systemic adjuvant (combined modality) therapy in the treatment of primary breast cancer, in: *Breast Cancer: Advances in Research and Treatment*, Vol. 1, *Current Approaches to Therapy* (W. L. McGuire, ed.), pp. 125–163, Plenum Press, New York (1977).
186. P. P. Carbone and D. C. Tormey, Combination chemotherapy for advanced disease, in: *Breast Cancer: Advances in Research and Treatment*, Vol. 1, *Current Approaches to Therapy* (W. L. McGuire, ed.), pp. 165–215, Plenum Press, New York (1977).
187. *The Breast Cancer Digest*, Office of Cancer Communications, National Cancer Institute, Bethesda, Maryland (1979).
188. R. Kushner, *Breast Cancer: A Personal History & an Investigative Report*, Harcourt Brace Jovanovich, New York (1975).
189. R. Kushner, Psyche and soma in breast disease, Panel discussion before the annual meeting of the American Psychological Association, Chicago (1976).
190. R. Kushner, Psychosocial aspects of breast cancer, in: *Psychosomatic Obstetrics and Gynecology* (D. D. Youngs and A. A. Ehrhardt, eds.), pp. 265–274, Appleton-Century-Crofts, New York (1979).
191. R. Kushner, The psychoemotional aspects of breast cancer, in: *A Sociological Framework for Patient Care*, 2nd ed. (J. R. Folta and E. S. Deck, eds.), pp. 379–392, John Wiley, New York, Chichester, Brisbane, Toronto (1979).
192. W. S. Schain, Guidelines for psychological management of breast cancer: A stage-related approach, in: *The Breast* (H. S. Gallager, ed.), pp. 465–475, C. V. Mosby, St. Louis (1978).
193. Gallup Organization, Inc., for the American Cancer Society, New York (1973).
194. B. F. Skinner, *Behavior of Organisms*, Appleton, New York (1938).
195. I. P. Pavlov, *Lectures on Conditioned Reflexes* (W. H. Gantt, transl.), International Publishers, New York (5th prntg.—1963).
196. J. W. Worden and A. D. Weisman, Psychososocial components of lagtime in cancer diagnosis, *J. Psychsom. Res.* **19**, 69–79 (1975).
197. A. D. Weisman and J. W. Worden, The existential plight in cancer: Significance of the first 100 days, *Int. J. Psychiatry Med.* **7**, 1–15 (1976).

198. M. Roach, Testimony presented before the Massachusetts Legislature in favor of the Patient's Rights Bill (February 1979).
199. J. Klemesrud, "Protestors assail refusal of Saks to hire woman after mastectomy," *New York Times*, March 25 (1977).
200. E. Kubler-Ross, *On Death and Dying*, Macmillan, New York (1969).
201. S. Stoddard, *The Hospice Movement*, Random House, New York (1978).
202. C. Saunders, *Care of the Dying*, Macmillan, London (1959).
203. M. J. Krant, *Dying and Dignity*, Charles C. Thomas, Springfield, Illinois (1974).

5

Breast Cancer Detection Center Projects

BENJAMIN FRANKLIN BYRD, JR.

1. Inception and Organization

During 1970, the medical leadership of the American Cancer Society studied available epidemiological data concerning cancer in the United States. It sought to evaluate the current position of the American Cancer Society in the ongoing fight against cancer, to develop special target areas for this fight, and to scrutinize the tools that were available to improve immediately the mortality from the leading types of cancer found in the United States.

Such a scrutiny had been made some years before when the society first entered into the area of early detection with its active support of the Papanicolau stain technique. Special utilization of the Pap smear for the detection of cancer of the reproductive tract had been selected as a major target area of the society. In large part, this activity had been the result of the efforts of Dr. Arthur Holleb and Dr. A. Hamblin Letton in developing a Task Force for Uterine Cancer Control. With the combination of early detection, good postnatal care, and definition and improvement of the methods of therapy currently available for uterine cancer, there was a drop in the incidence and death rate from cancer of the cervix and corpus uteri.[1] This work dropped cancer of the uterus from the principal cause of cancer death in women to a very modest role as a contributing factor in the continuing death rate from cancer in women.[2]

On scrutiny of the epidemiological figures available in 1970, it became obvious that breast cancer in women of the United States was of epidemic proportions. At the time of that study, it was evident that 1 of

---

BENJAMIN FRANKLIN BYRD, JR. • Nashville, Tennessee 37203.

every 15 women in the United States would develop breast cancer at some point during her life. There had been no objective improvement in mortality from breast cancer during the 40 years prior to 1970. The great majority of women who presented themselves for therapy were coming in at a comparatively late date in the natural history of their disease. The cancers were being picked up predominantly by the women themselves. This detection was not accomplished through any concerted effort at breast self-examination, but because of a simple physical mass that attracted the attention of the patient. Because of these facts, the Senior Vice President for Medical Affairs of the American Cancer Society, Dr. Arthur Holleb, convened the "Action and Planning Committee on Breast Cancer Control" of the American Cancer Society. This committee was charged to study the ability of the society to intervene directly in the breast-cancer problem in such a fashion that a significant improvement in the mortality of those women who were discovered to have breast cancer could be effected. As a matter of policy, the society does not intervene in the therapy of the individual patients. The general effort of the society was toward early detection of breast cancer with earlier intervention in the natural history of the cancer.

It is a well-established fact that the natural history of breast cancer prior to the tumor's reaching its physically detectable size (1 cm in diameter) requires at least 20 doubling times, and from one cell to 1 mm in diameter 10 more doubling times, a total of 30 doubling times from one cell to 1 cm *if all cells divide and survive.*[3] (See Fig. 1).

All available information at the time of the original meeting of the Cancer Control Committee (later to be known as the Task Force for Breast Cancer Control) showed a definite relationship between the frequency with which metastatic disease was found in the axillary lumph nodes and the size of the primary tumor at the time of initial therapy (see Appendix I). With the information that was available, this gave real hope that by early intervention the disease could be treated at an earlier clinical stage, so that with intervention at an earlier stage of favorable alteration in "cure rate" might reasonably be expected.

At the first meeting of the Breast Cancer Control Group of the American Cancer Society, the discussion was quite broad in its extent. There were a series of factors that offered material hope of improving at

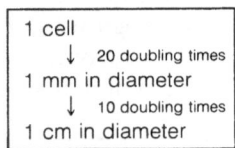

Fig. 1. Breast cancer growth rate (if all cells divide and survive).

least the survival with breast cancer. A possibility was offered of favorably altering the incidence of breast cancer. These facts were (1) the known high occurrence rate of cancer of the breast in women of America and western Europe; (2) the knowledge also available of the relatively low incidence of breast cancer in Oriental groups; (3) the fact that the single biggest predictor in the incidence of cancer of the breast is the age of the patient. While cancer of the breast is the most common cause of death in women between 35 and 44 years of age, it becomes an increasingly more frequent disease until age 80, when its proportional incidence level becomes constant. Comparison of the incidence figures of breast cancer in the Westernized civilizations and in developing countries gives evidence that there are two different types of breast cancer, one type occurring before age 50 and a second[4] type that accounts for the major incidence of breast cancer in Western women occurring after age 50. There is a similar rise in incidence in the developing nations for which statistical documentation is available.[4]

Besides the evidence related to the natural history and incidence of cancer, the role of X-ray examination of the breast (mammography) was poorly defined. It seemed that with this technique, there were great expectations for developing an early diagnostic procedure for breast cancer. This was particularly borne out in the Health Insurance Plan study, which will be discussed in detail a little later.[5] It has been shown that in some cancer there is an increased skin temperature in the overlying skin. This led to the utilization of thermographic studies with the idea that temperature variations might offer "early detection" at an early clinical or preclinical level.

There seemed little doubt to the group that available information about breast self-examination was being poorly disseminated. Although the American Cancer Society had made concerted efforts to interest women of the United States in breast self-examination, the great majority of women who were at risk from breast cancer were not making use of this very valuable self-help program.

The role of the society in improving treatment of the patient with breast cancer seemed to be twofold: (1) to develop new techniques by laboratory and clinical investigation that would permit more effective ablation of early breast cancer and (2) to make available to the medical population generally the advances in breast-cancer management that permitted both early detection and adequate treatment suited to the needs of the patient. For this purpose, the society created its Task Force for Breast Cancer Control (see Appendix I), which the writer chaired at its inception in February 1972. At that time, the Task Force was composed of specialists in the several disciplines intimately associated with the breast-cancer problem. There were physicians who were involved in family practice, surgery, diagnostic radiology, pathology, and gynecology, as well as various members of the staff of the American Cancer Society with special expertise in epidemiology. There were also women consumers present as advisors. It was the opinion of this group that the society could support, for a period of two years, 12 Breast Cancer Detection Demonstration Projects (BCDDPs). It would be the purpose of these projects to demonstrate the capacity for the early detection of breast cancer by obtaining from each participant in the demonstration project a history of problems relating to breast cancer by physical examination done by physicians or by specially trained allied health personnel, by a thermographic examination of the breasts of the participants, by mammographic examination of the breasts, and by educating the participant in breast self-examination. It seemed wise to place the projects in a diverse group of professional environments such as university hospitals, community facilities, major metropolitan hospitals, and specialized institutes with a particular interest in breast cancer. Not an inconsiderable aspect of the planning at this stage was the ability of the American Cancer Society to finance these centers. It is of interest that the direct financial contribution of the American Cancer Society alone in this program eventually reached an $8-million-plus level.

The "Conquest of Cancer" Act had been passed by Congress in 1971, about the same time that the society expressed its interest in breast-cancer control in concrete form. This "Conquest of Cancer" Act directed the head of the National Cancer Institute (NCI) to "establish programs as necessary for cooperation with state and other health agencies in the diagnosis, prevention, and treatment of cancer."[6] An invitation was extended by the American Cancer Society to the NCI in March 1972 (see Appendix II) to collaborate in the BCDDP effort. These projects provided a particular opportunity to work out a cooperative effort between the Federal government and the private sector. Dr. Frank Rauscher, then Director of the NCI, entered into an agreement with the American Cancer Society that made it possible to increase the BCDDPs to a nationwide scope with 27 centers being created (see Appendix III). Each of these centers was to examine an unchanging population group of 10,000 women annually for a period of five examinations. The direct supervisory authority for the NCI was given to Dr. Nathaniel I. Berlin.

The decision on selection of population groups for the projects was debated rather generally by the staffs of both the NCI and the American Cancer Society. A special point was made that since breast cancer was the leading cause of death of women between 35 and 44 years of age, early detection in this group was especially important. The lower limit of the selection group was then placed at 35. The upper limit was placed at 74 for a variety of reasons related to cooperation and ability to participate as well as the high incidence of breast cancer in the older age groups. There was grave doubt about the ability of the projects to enlist the support of women in the communities, and one of the specific tasks assigned to the American Cancer Society was the use of its volunteers in getting a broad-based representation among study groups in the various concerned communities. The women who participated were self-selected. Built into the original protocols were commitments to involve minority-group enrollees. Many of the same problems were encountered in enlisting minority-group representation that have so often surfaced in other self-selected health-care programs. This motivation to self-selection resulted in a group of women entering the study group who were possibly at special risk. The presence of a positive family history, the presence of previous breast disease, and the presence of a suspected lesion in the enrollee's breast were all things that might cause a woman to pursue this opportunity to have repeated careful breast examinations at no dollar cost to her. This self-selection did not interfere at all with the purpose of the demonstration projects, which was to demonstrate the capability for early detection of breast cancer. If it had been possible to restrict the role of the projects to those women who would at some time in the near present or distant future develop breast cancer, it would have been well suited to the capability of the techniques in the project to detect breast cancer at an early stage, to see what the results of treatment of breast cancer at this early stage were, and to follow these women for the period of five repeated examinations and for 10 years' follow-up to determine the effect on their future life and life expectancy. It was not a study of incidence but a study of the capability of several techniques devised to bring about early detection of breast cancer. As an adjunct to early detection, it would evaluate early surgical intervention and the ability of surgical intervention to alter long-term survival rates.

There were six objectives entered into by the American Cancer Society and the NCI, and these were listed in March 1973 as follows[7]:

1. To find whether the methods for detection of breast cancer could be applied to the general population through regular medical channels.
2. To determine whether a negative thermogram is sufficient to preclude the use of clinical examination and mammography in the detection of breast cancer.
3. To determine whether volunteers could bring in an adequate number of women for screening and provide follow-up. These volunteers would also help staff the project offices, a demonstration of community spirit that also reduced cost considerably.

4. To determine whether nonpalpable breast cancer properly treated would provide more years free of cancer than waiting for palpable evidence of disease.
5. To evaluate the effect of literature on the teaching of breast self-examination and to determine whether women continue breast self-examination and, if they do not, why not.
6. To try to better define those women at high risk for breast cancer.

Subsequently, these goals were expanded in January 1974 to include studies on demography and on the role and effectiveness of public and professional education. The professional aspects of the evaluation of the tumors picked up in the demonstration projects were thought to include an increase in the use of specimen radiography and a pathological evaluation of the size of the cancer itself, of the histological structure of the cancer, and of the presence of axillary node metastases. The results of treatment were used in appraising the benefits of early detection. These special interests resulted in great emphasis on the role of the pathologist in evaluating the specimens that were removed, and this emphasis on pathological study has been implemented largely through the efforts of Dr. William Hartmann and his Pathology Study Group. This study is continuing.

When these programs became available across the country, they were well publicized through the leading lay and medical journals. The total enrollment of 280,000 women was rapidly achieved. There was a consistent distribution throughout the centers that was remarkable in that in the total group, about 50% of the women were 35–49 years of age at enrollment, and 50% of the group were 50–74 years of age. By the time the results of the examinations of the first 50,000 women were available, a few constant patterns were found that have persisted throughout the entire study. The figures showed that about one third of the cancers occurred in that 50% of the group that were between 35 and 49 years of age at the time they entered the program, while two thirds of the cancers found were in the group of women between 50 and 74 years of age when they entered the study.[8]

2. Second Thoughts

Two events took place that modified the course of the Breast Cancer Detection Demonstration Projects (BCDDPs) quite dramatically. The first was the personal experience of the wives of the President and the Vice President of the United States, Mrs. Gerald Ford and Mrs. Nelson Rockefeller. Both these ladies developed breast cancer in a fairly brief

period of time. These two very fine women spoke out most courageously about their experience with breast cancer and reemphasized the
problem to all American women. This event brought an increased en-
thusiasm for participation in the BCDDPs, as well as a marked increase
in public interest in the early detection and management of breast
cancer.

The second thing that materially altered the course of the BCDDPs
was the extrapolation by some epidemiologists of presumptive risks (see
Appendix IV) of X-ray examination of the breast. This came from the
experience with the Hiroshima and Nagasaki bomb blasts and from
certain instances of the use of therapeutic radiation.[9] The extrapolation
was based on doses that were a great deal higher than the exposure that
resulted from screening and from diagnostic mammography. The exposure involved in any of these experiences as well as the data base for any
of these extrapolations was far higher than the average exposure in the
American Cancer Society–National Cancer Institute BCDDPs. Those
who believed that such a linear extrapolation existed pointed out that
from these very high doses of radiation, it might be deduced that even 1
rad of diagnostic radiation might slightly increase the risk that breast
cancer will develop many years later.[10] Casual remarks were made
about inducing epidemics of breast cancer, yet even the most vigorous
review cannot substantiate a scientific base for that observation. The
experience of Mrs. Ford and Mrs. Rockefeller increased public anxiety
about breast cancer. The remarks of those who emphasized the risk of
radiation exposure increased the anxiety about early diagnosis. These
two sources of anxiety created a difficult dichotomy, at best.

3. The Beahrs Report

In 1975, the National Cancer Institute (NCI) reviewed the rising
estimates of presumptive risks of radiation exposure given during
screening or mammography for breast cancer. The NCI at that time
asked Dr. Oliver Beahrs, who was chief of the surgical section at Mayo
Clinic, to review the available data from the BCDDPs. To achieve this end,
three committees were appointed: a clinical group chaired by Dr. Charles
Smartt, an epidemiological and biostatistical group chaired by Mr. Sam
Shapiro, and at a somewhat later date, a pathological review group chaired
by Dr. Robert McDivett. The review was restricted to the data available
through June 13, 1976, and included the group of women who had had
both a first and second screening achieved by the cutoff date, June 30, 1976.
The report of the "Beahrs Committee"[8] was received at a consensus
development meeting on breast-cancer screening that was held in 1977

at the National Institutes of Health, and this marked essentially a mid-point review of the data available through the BCDDPs (Table I). The general clinical results that were reported by Dr. Smartt's clinical study group at this meeting showed that in the first BCDDP screen, there were 261,859 women, and in the second screen, 146,364 at the time of the report. In this group, there were 734 cancers found through recommended biopsies, 109 in the early-recall group, and 145 "interval cases." At the time of the second screening, the corresponding figures were 232 at the second 12-month examination, 15 in the early-recall group, and 73 "interval cases" during the second 12 months. In the first-screen cohort, there were found 516 infiltrating cancers, and 51% of these under 1 cm were detected by mammography. Since the tumors were larger at the time they came to definitive therapy, more of the tumors had been picked up by physical examination or by patient detection. In this original group, 43.9% were diagnosed by mammography alone, 47.7% were detected by both mammography and physical examination, and 7.4% were evident on physical examination alone with no mammographic evidence of neoplasm. Thermography proved to be very disappointing and was felt to have, for the general purposes of the BCDDPs, no value as part of the detection program.

The report of the Beahrs committee, particularly relating to radiation exposure, the risk of later breast cancer as a result of the radiation exposure, and the value of mammography, was generally discussed. The value of the detection program was unfortunately passed over after a relatively brief review in the press because of some arguments that arose about the clinical management of the cancers that were picked up as a product of the demonstration projects. The demonstration projects are not now and were never intended to dictate therapy. They were, from the earliest days, charged with accumulating information about the results of the form of treatment that was employed, but they did not dictate any protocols for management of patients with breast cancer once the cancers had been identified by biopsy.

Table I
Biopsies Reported

Time of examination	Benign	Aspiration	Cancer	Malignant (%)
1st Year	7,688	665	1499	17.9
Recall	2,372	278	274	10.3
TOTALS	10,050	943	1773	16.1

4. The Course of Events

One of the most difficult chores related to the BCDDPs was evaluation of data generated by the project. This was done under contract with the University City Science Center Data Management Center in Philadelphia. Dr. George Foradori served as the Data Management Officer and did an excellent job of getting the data submitted from the demonstration projects into an assimilable form. There have been innumerable conflicts in the time and method of reporting from the various data centers. Most of these have been resolved as of October 1979. Instead of new problems arising daily, they now occur at about weekly intervals. The latest material available extends through February 28, 1979, and is shown in Table II.[11]

The recall examinations included are made up of those individuals concerning whom a definitive decision could not be made at the time of the annual examination. These individuals were brought back at an interval of from 1 to 11 months prior to the next annual examination. The figures are still unedited for the current status of the various programs, but it now seems that there were 273,108 women enrolled originally in the BCDDPs, as shown in Table III. This has not changed in the last five months and is not likely to change, except for some editorial corrections. In the group of enrollees at the original examination, there were 10,412 biopsies recommended on the basis of the original evaluation. During the first year after the initial examination, but prior to the second annual examination, there were 40,736 women reexamined, and of these 3419 had biopsies recommended as a result of changes on either X-ray or

Table II
Current Status of Programs

Time of examination	Through February 28, 1979	Biopsies recorded
1st Year	273,108	10,412
Recall	40,736	3,419
2nd Year	235,345	5,265
Recall	13,572	1,379
3rd Year	205,124	4,006
Recall	10,311	1,097
4th Year	159,974	2,897
Recall	6,347	702
5th Year	65,184	1,080
Recall	2,008	198
TOTALS	1,011,709	30,455

Table III
Detection Mammography[a]

	"Suspicious malignant"	
Examination	Mammography	Physical examination
1st exam	2%	0.7%
Subsequent exams	1%	0.2%

[a]One third of examinations showed some abnormality.

physical examination. At the time of this report, 235,345 women had returned for the second annual examination. A total of 5265 biopsies were recommended at the time of the second annual examination. This figure has not changed except for some editorial corrections in the past five months, so it too may be accepted as essentially a final figure.

Of the women in the original group, 13.8% dropped out during the first year. There was a marked drop in the number of recall examinations during the second 12 months. This might have been anticipated, since the difficult cases were winnowed out during the first 2 years. One of every ten women who were recalled had biopsies recommended at the time of recall examination. At the first examination, 4% of the population group had a biopsy recommended, and at the second 12-month examination, fewer than 2% were recommended to have biopsies.

At the third 12-month examination, the dropouts increased to 25% of the original enrollees. Again, this figure will not apparently be greatly altered by additional accumulation of information, since there has been minimal, only editorial change in this figure in the past five months. It was recommended in 2% of the women examined at the third 12-month examination that biopsies be carried out. At the recall examinations following the third 12-month examination, 10,311 women were examined and 10% were recommended to have follow-up examinations.

In looking at the first 3 years, the dropout attrition rate may be attributed to a great many things. Of major significance was the widespread publicity given concerning the risk of mammography. There have been some population shifts. There was almost certainly a lack of interest after a negative first examination. On the other hand, the presence of anxiety about a cancer being picked up may have caused some women not to return. In the most effective of the demonstration projects, the dropout rate was around 15%. The highest attrition rate was in the large metropolitan areas, where the dropout rate was as high as 50%.

The fourth and fifth 12-month examination figures are growing with each passing month. The Seattle program has closed down and has completed its final examinations. On a percentage basis, the proportion of biopsies recommended at both the fourth and fifth 12-month examinations and at the recalls during these periods remains essentially the same as the earlier examinations. One of the remarkable things about the whole program has been the consistency of the significant figures since its earliest examinations. There is available a data base for the demonstration projects of over a million examinations and records of 30,455 biopsies that have been recommended.

One of every three examinations at the initial evaluation showed some abnormality. The lesions were graded relatively as malignant, "suspicious malignant," "suspicious benign," or "negative." Of those examinations that were rated either malignant or "suspicious malignant" on mammography, 2% of the total population group was felt to have a "suspicious malignant" lesion. On the original physical examination, 0.7% of the population group was felt to have a "suspicious malignant" lesion. At subsequent examinations, this figure dropped to 1% on mammography and 0.2% on physical evaluation, as shown in Table III. These changes represent the difference between prevalence and incidence. Using the Surveillance Epidemiology and End Results Program (SEER) figures for anticipated incidence of breast cancer in a group of women in the United States of the ages entered in this group, it was estimated that there would be two cancers per thousand enrollees per year in women of the ages entered in the BCDDPs. So far during the first 12 months, there have been found 1773 cancers in the group of 273,108 examinees. This is a figure of 6.5 cases per thousand women examined during the first 12 months of the program. This is essentially the prevalence of carcinoma of the breast in the group evaluated, and it is about 3 times the incidence anticipated in this group. At subsequent examinations, the incidence figures anticipated from the SEER report have been accurately reproduced in the cancer detected from biopsies recommended by the BCDDPs.

The number of aspirations carried out is interesting, since these represent means of avoiding incisional biopsy. With very few exceptions, the diagnosis of cancer has been confirmed by biopsy, so that those individuals who have a positive diagnosis of cancer have an incisional biopsy to confirm that observation. The current totals of diagnostic procedures are indicative of the experience in those individuals who were subjected to further diagnostic procedures on the basis of a rec-

Table IV
Current Totals: Diagnostic Procedures[a]

Cases	Benign	Aspiration	Cancer	Total
Number	22,358	4103	3788	30,249
Percentage of total	73.9	13.6	12.5	100

[a]Of the biopsies, cancer represents 16.9%.

ommendation from the BCDDP. The total of 30,249 individuals in whom either an aspiration or incisional biopsy was recommended resulted in 73.9% benign diagnoses; 13.6% were treated by aspiration and 12.5% were found to have cancer. Of the biopsies, it should be emphasized that those individuals who had a suspicious lesion on aspiration were then subjected to incisional biopsy. Of the biopsies, 16.9% contained cancer when examined by the pathologists. Table IV summarizes these totals.

The pathology review will be discussed in Section 6, but it is interesting to put the results of the biopsies in the proper frame of reference. Of those biopsies that are reported and are reviewed, 85% were benign, 14% showed an invasive carcinoma, and 1% showed preinvasive carcinoma or carcinoma *in situ*, as illustrated in Table V. Here we must grapple with the new concept of minimal cancers. Dr. Richard Coslow has shown that in a preliminary evaluation of the program's data for the modality of detection of the reported cancers (shown in Table VI), 45% of the cancers found in the demonstration projects were found on mammography alone. These cancers were associated with a negative physical examination. In 42% of the patients who had cancers, there were changes both on mammography and on physical examination. These dual pieces of evidence were the indication for biopsy. There were 6% of the patients who had no change on mammography on which surgical intervention could be recommended, yet this 6% had some physical changes that brought about a biopsy recommendation from the BCDDP. Of the cancers, 7% were found without any change

Table V
Biopsies Reported
and Reviewed

85%	Benign
14%	Invasive cancer
1%	Preinvasive or *in situ* cancer

Table VI
Preliminary Analysis of
Progress Data:
Modality Results for Cancers
Reported

Modality[b]	Percentage of total cancers
M+ P −	45
M+ P+	42
M − P+	6
M − P −	7
	100%

[a]Period covered: start through December 1977.
[b]Where all modalities were performed and reported and age group is known. (M) Mammography; (P) physical examination.

either on mammogram or on physical examination. These tumors were found in a variety of fashions, some on so-called prophylactic mastectomy. Cancers were discovered in some instances as the result of elective surgery, of reduction or augmentation mammoplasty, or of a blind biopsy of the opposite side. Pathological examination of the tissues that were removed in conjunction with these procedures showed a carcinoma.

There was in the later 12-month examinations a group of patients who presented themselves for the 12-month examination, but did not recieve a mammographic exam. This might have been the result of the anxiety arising from the widespread discussions of the risk of mammography or as a result of the administration's decision to limit the mammographic examination in women under 50. It was the right of any patient in the program to refuse any part of the evaluation, but generally there were a significant number of refusals only in the area of mammography.

Table VII shows that at the time of the first evaluation, 99.3% of the examinees had mammograms done and 2.4% of these were interpreted as being malignant or "suspicious malignant." There had been very little public impact from the discussion of the radiation risk of mammography at the time of the second examination, and 94% of the examinees had mammographic examination and 1.3% of the examinations were read as "suspicious malignant." By the time of the third 12-month examination, there had been fairly wide dissemination both of the alteration in

Table VII
Significance of Omitted Mammographic Examinations

Year of examination	Number of examinees	Number of mammograms[a]	Number of suspicious malignant[b]
1st	273,108	271,095 (99.3%)	6195 (2.4%)
2nd	235,345	220,181 (94.0%)	2814 (1.3%)
3rd	205,124	153,648 (74.9%)	1838 (1.2%)
4th	159,974	100,347 (62.1%)	1359 (1.3%)
5th	65,184	42,172 (64.7%)	632 (1.4%)

[a]In parentheses are the percentages of total examinees having mammograms.
[b]In parentheses are the percentages of mammograms interpreted as malignant or suspicious malignant.

guidelines for the examinees and of the aroused public anxiety about radiation exposure. The number of examinees having mammograms at the third 12-month examination dropped to 74.9%. Of the 153,648 women who underwent mammography, 1838, or 1.2%, were found to have lesions that were "suspicious malignant." The fourth- and fifth-year groups are not yet complete. We do find that the number of women having mammograms is down to 62 and 64% respectively, yet the number of "suspicious malignant" lesions has remained essentially constant at 1.3 and 1.4%. The women in the third, fourth, and fifth 12-month examination groups who had mammograms were selected either because they were at special risk or because they were in the older age groups. It is amazing that in this group of women, the percentage of "suspicious malignant" mammographic studies has remained constant. This can only lead to the observation that it sould be equally constant in the group of women who were not examined. It is not unreasonable to assume that in the more than one hundred thousand women on whom mammograms were not done at the third, fourth, and fifth examinations, there would be the same incidence of cancer as there was in the group on whom these examinations were done with a "suspicious malignant" rate of 1.2%. This seems like a very high price to pay for the anxiety connected with the radiation exposure from mammography. We are indebted to Brinton et al. [12] for the excellent review of the relative risk factors in terms of multiples of control-group risks (Table VIII). There is a definite increase in risk in the women with a weight over 155 pounds, with more than one previous biopsy, and with an age of 30 or more at the birth of the first child. The most significant finding seems to be the importance of the family history of breast cancer, which is higher with the grandmother than with the mother because there is still a long time lag in many of these women during which the mother may develop

Table VIII
Relative Risks

Risk factor	Relative risk[a]
Weight of 155 lbs or more	1.51
More than one previous breast biopsy	2.05
Age of 30 or more at first birth	2.15
Family history of breast cancer	
Mother	3.88
Grandmother	4.82
Mother and grandmother	4.87

[a]In multiples of control-group risk.

her breast cancer. In those women who are under 50 years of age with a maternal familial history of breast cancer, there is more than a 6-fold increase in the risk of developing breast cancer over the risk of their sister population.

5. Follow-up

The issues that arose from the Breast Cancer Detection Demonstration Projects (BCDDPs) became quite obvious as the projects began to reach the end of their five 12-month examinations. A review committee under the co-chairmanship of Dr. Larry H. Baker and Dr. Gerald Metter was formed.[13] Serving with these were representatives of the statistical study group and of the BCDDPs. In favor of a 5-year annual follow-up on all screenees were that:

1. All screenees have contracted for and are expected to participate in the 5-year follow-up program.
2. There was an opportunity for studying the impact of a major screening program if a complete data set was available for all the examinees.
3. Should adverse effects appear, there would be continuing contact with the total population of screenees.

These factors were offset by the facts that:

1. There was a limited amount of scientific information available on screenees. This was due to the absence of a specific hypothesis that had been set forth by the original enrollment schedule.
2. There would be a major dollar expenditure in following these 280,000 women, and the major portion of this information could

be obtained by following all the cancers and all the biopsies performed or recommended with matched controls from the group
of examinees.

3. It is generally acknowledged that a 5-year follow-up of all women
   enrolled in the projects would not yield any new information
   about radiation risk.

The subcommittee recommended the creation of a case control triad
with an effort to identify the risk factors for breast cancer that might be
demonstrable within the group reviewed in the BCDDPs. This would
result in some expansion of the material that was available on the original enrollment questionnaires, particularly in relation to menopausal
estrogens, oral contraceptives, antihypertensives, and other drugs. This
triad was to be:

1. All the breast-cancer cases that were known to have occurred in
   the BCDDP participants.
2. A matched case with a noncancer biopsy for each breast-cancer
   case.
3. A matched screenee with no biopsy recommended for each
   breast-cancer case.

As closely as possible, these were to be matched by age, race, screening
project, demonstration project, and the annual examination at which the
matched case was identified. It was hoped that:

1. This would reveal variations in characteristics of the women who
   persisted in the program for as many as four or five 12-month
   reexaminations.
2. The cases that developed later in the screening examination
   might show some biological differentiation from the cases that
   dominated the early examinations.
3. The data base would play a major role in the plans for the projected follow-up projects.

It was recognized that the group would have a relatively small
number of "events" during the first 5-year follow-up, but perhaps
within the numbers involved it would be possible to identify areas that
deserve continuing examination.

Still another alternative was to examine the triad of women plus all
the women who had noncancer biopsies and in addition normal controls
matched to this group. It was the opinion of the subcommittee that an
exit interview should be done so that the women would know that they
have been selected for follow-up and the opportunity be given to emphasize the importance of their cooperation. In addition, information

was obtained from each woman that would facilitate a 5-year follow-up, in particular her Social Security number, her husband, name changes, and her maiden name.

It was recommended by the subcommittee that this follow-up of the triad plus all biopsies and matched controls represented the most effective use of the material available through the BCDDPs. This recommendation was made to the National Cancer Advisory Board, and was approved by them in due time.

On the basis of the recommendation from the National Cancer Advisory Board, the National Cancer Institute, in June 1979, started to issue contracts to carry out the recommended follow-up. It was the intent of the contract that this follow-up would include all the women enrolled in the BCDDPs who had a biopsy carried out, whether this biopsy was recommended by the BCDDP or not. These women will be matched to a control group. A second group includes those women who had a biopsy recommended but in whom the biopsy was not carried out. The object of this is to evaluate the screening programs for their impact on both the screenee and the health-delivery system, with special consideration for the goals of the BCDDPs.

The second major goal of the follow-up was to determine the issues in detection, etiology, and natural history of breast disease. This was to be accomplished by special study of:

1. All cancers detected by modalities within the screening program.
2. Cancers in BCDDP participants not detected in the screening program.
3. A screened population with biopsy recommended but not performed.
4. A screened population with biopsies performed but not recommended.
5. Special pathological subtypes of cancer with emphasis on carcinoma *in situ* and invasive carcinoma less than 1 cm in diameter.
6. Pathological subtypes of duct, atypia, and other graduations of benign breast disease.
7. Screened women with benign breast disease documented by mammography or physical examination only.
8. Screened women without breast disease as documented by mammography and physical examination over a 5-year period.
9. Screened women with specific abnormal thermographic patterns.
10. Screened women with specific demographic risk factors.

To accomplish this, it is the intent of the contract with the various BCDDPs that women be interviewed annually on approximately the anniversary date of their entry into the project. Once entered as a part of the follow-up, each woman selected must be followed and must be accounted for. This is an integral part of the interview and of the conduct of the program itself. It is the intent of the program that if all else fails, she is to be followed through the National Cancer for Health Statistics, National Death Index, using her Social Security number. This is to be done only as a last resort. There will be four study-group assignments:

Group I. Cancers: This group includes both project-recommended and potential interval cancers.

Group II. Benign biopsies/aspirations: As in Group I, this group includes biopsies and aspirations recommended by the project as well as those that were performed without a specific project recommendation (that is, potential interval surgery).

Group III. Normals: Women who had no surgery or recommendation for surgical consultation (biopsy or aspiration) during the screening or "project normals." A woman who had breast surgery prior to entering the screening project could still be a "project normal."

Group IV. Surgical consultations recommended by the project but not performed: This group includes participants who had recommendation for either biopsy or aspiration.

Once a woman has entered the follow-up, she will remain in the group to which she was originally assigned although her status may change. The material accumulated from these follow-ups is to be handled through the Data Management Center in Philadelphia, as were the general figures that were generated by the BCDDPs. This follow-up is now under way by contract in at least two of the projects. It is anticipated that as the other projects become eligible, the opportunity will be extended to them to participate in the continuing follow-up.

6. Pathology Review

At the time that the Breast Cancer Detection Demonstration Projects (BCDDPs) were conceived, the significance of relative homogeneous pathology data was recognized. To this end, each project had a project pathologist, who was responsible for coordinating the activities of the demonstration projects with the hospitals in the community. There was no treatment protocol involved in the demonstration project outlines. It was realized that each of the enrollees for whom biopsy was recommended would have to seek, through the health-care facilities that were available, a suitable treatment on the basis of the recommendation of the BCDDP. Retrieval of the data from the biopsies and aspirations as well as retrieval of information about the actual treatment protocol of those individuals who were found to have cancer was an extremely difficult task. It involved a high degree of cooperation from the pathologists in the community, and this, of course, was greatly upset by the remarks generated in the Beahrs report. These remarks created a difficult atmosphere for the project pathologists. This has been only partially ameliorated by the continuing efforts of the College of American Pathologists and the various pathologists who were intimately involved in the BCDDPs.

In 1975, it became obvious that it was necessary to accomplish some review of the diagnoses that were rendered by the project pathologists as well as the hospital pathologists. This recognition resulted in the creation of a Pathology Quality Control Program. This program, funded in 1976, divided the programs in the country into eight regions with a regional pathologist responsible for reviewing the pathological material generated by no fewer than three, nor more than five, of the projects. It also created a Central Review Group (or a Central Advisory Group) that was given the final responsibility for classifying material from any patient in the BCDDP and the responsibility for monitoring the Pathology Control Program. After three years, this control program was reviewed independently, and it seemed wise to terminate the regional review system. This resulted in the material's being forwarded directly from the project pathologist to the Central Repository in the Department of Pathology at Vanderbilt University Medical Center. Concurrence between the pathologist of the Central Repository (Vanderbilt Center) and the project pathologists was recorded as per the diagnosis of the project pathologist.

Any nonconcurrence at any level or any questionable diagnosis was reviewed by a Central Advisory Group consisting of Drs. Stephen Gallagher, William Hartmann, Robert V. P. Hutter, Harold Oberman, and Paul Peter Rosen. It is the function of this group to review and resolve the nonconcurrence with the project pathologist.

Accumulation of data from the doctors' offices or the approximately 7000 acute-care hospitals in this country has been very complex. For instance, it has been a real chore to notify the hospital pathologist that a given patient who has undergone surgical treatment of her breast is a patient in one of the BCDDPs. It is then necessary to obtain the material from the hospital pathologist, review the material, and return a concurrence or nonconcurrence for the notification of the hospital pathologist.

For the purposes of classification, the Central Advisory Committee deals with only three categories: (1) benign; (2) *in situ* carcinoma; and (3)

170	Benjamin Franklin Byrd, Jr.

invasive carcinoma. There are two indeterminate groups: (1) between benign and malignant and (2) between *in situ* and invasive carcinoma.

The review program of the Pathology Quality Control is based entirely on the pathological material available. The Quality Control Group does not have available to it any of the other material concerning the enrollee under study. The report of the Pathology Quality Control Program at the end of 1979[14] revealed that there were, at that time, nine cases of possible nonconcurrence in the entire program. This represented 6008 cases reviewed to that date. Three of these were called carcinoma at the project level (one invasive, two *in situ*), whereas the Control Advisory Group classified these benign—a possible positive nonconcurrence rate of 0.05%. There were six cases classified as *in situ* carcinoma by the Central Advisory Group that had been called benign by the project pathologist—this giving a negative nonconcurrence rate of 0.1%. It is of special interest that there were no cases classified as invasive carcinoma by the Control Advisory Group that had been called benign by the project pathologist. This gives real evidence of the high level of diagnostic credibility for breast-cancer disease among the pathologists. These observations serve in large part to offset the unfavorable comments that arose following the Beahrs report, which was the first analytical survey of material available through the BCDDPs.

7. Conclusion

The history of the Breast Cancer Detection Demonstration Projects (BCDDPs) is not yet complete. Some of the projects are still winding down the fifth and final evaluation of the enrollees. The termination of the project will occur only when the last of the projected follow-up is accomplished. At that time, a more critical review of its impact will be practical.

For the time being, one must look at the six projected goals that were established in 1973 by the American Cancer Society and the National Cancer Institute. These are outlined in Section 1:

1. The methods employed in the BCDDPs have resulted in detection of breast cancer earlier in the biological history of the disease. The techniques that were employed in the survey can be adapted through regular medical channels to detection of breast cancer. It is a source of some regret that no new techniques have come into common use during the seven years that have elapsed since the initiation of the program.

2. The role of the thermogram is not clearly defined. It is evident that thermography is a substitute neither for clinical examination nor for

radiographic examination in the detection of breast cancer. Its clinical reliability seems to still be limited to a few unusually capable centers, and it has no application, in the experience of the BCDDPs, as a screening technique.

3. The volunteers of the American Cancer Society, with a tremendous demonstration of community spirit, have been able to involve women as enrollees in the BCDDPs. The volunteers had an active part in the follow-up of enrollees, and all these efforts have resulted in the much lower cost to the sources of financing for the BCDDPs.

4. The initial findings of the pathology review of those individuals who had their cancers picked up in the BCDDP have shown clear evidence that the cancers detected have been at a biologically earlier date than those that were commonly encountered in practice prior to 1973. Not enough time has yet elapsed to make it clear and confirmable that patients in whom this earlier intervention has been possible will have the expected survival benefits that ordinarily go along with detection of breast cancer before the presence of axillary nodes is demonstrable. This is an indication of the fairly brief duration of the study, rather than the product of any identifiable doubt that the projected benefits will not be realized.

5. The public-education aspects of the BCDDPs have been enormous. The emergence of the BCDDPs followed closely the increased public awareness of breast cancer. It now seems that 9% of the women of the United States will develop breast cancer at some time in their lives. This figure has increased in the past ten years. Public awareness has led and will undoubtedly continue to lead to increased consciousness of the necessity for new techniques for detection and for new and appropriate methods of managing the individual who has a carcinoma of the breast. Breast self-examination is a well-known, well-publicized, and acknowledged part of the existence of most mature and well-informed women in the United States.

6. Great steps forward have been taken in identifying those women who are at high risk for breast cancer. The clear parameters of risk are related to a maternal familial history or an individual history of breast cancer. The somewhat lower risk associated with benign breast diseases gives some assurance to the many women who have undergone treatment for mammary dysplasia. Breast cancer screening by the techniques of the BCDDPs would be most usable if some identification of a high risk segment of the female population were possible. It was the hope of the original programmers that approximately 25% of the total female population could be identified by history or physical markers as being at special risk. In this relatively small segment of the population, it was

projected that up to 90% of all breast cancers would occur. Identification of such a small, major risk group has not been possible from data so far available.

The impact of breast cancer in the United States will be appreciably ameliorated by the experience of the demonstration projects and the public and professional education that have been an integral part of their course. We all look forward to seeing an ultimate evaluation of the fruits of this experience. Every cooperation must continue between the American Cancer Society and the National Cancer Institute as well as the various BCDDPs to make available to the public the wealth of information that has been gleaned and to identify the fruits of this data base to those worldwide population groups that are at major risk, and especially to the women of the United States.

Appendix I

Report of Action and Planning Committee on Breast Cancer Control
to the
Medical and Scientific Executive Committee

November 2, 1971

At the Survey Committee meeting held in New York City on September 7 and 8, 1971, Dr. Holleb made a presentation on the current magnitude of the breast cancer problem. It was pointed out that breast cancer remains the number 1 killer of women; that one of every 15 newborn girls may be expected to develop breast cancer at some time during their lives; that one woman dies of breast cancer every 15–20 minutes while 3 more women are being diagnosed as having breast cancer in that same time interval and that there has not been a significant change in the mortality rate of breast cancer in the past 35 years. Other data were used to reinforce the concept that education of the public about breast self-examination and periodic health examinations, as well as professional education programs should be expanded, but that these alone may not be enough to markedly alter the number of deaths from breast cancer. Newer techniques like mammography, thermography and other modalities were mentioned as possible avenues toward the earlier detection of breast cancer—detection at a stage described as "minimal breast cancer." The Survey Committee asked Dr. Holleb to organize a committee of experts to review the problem and called on Dr. George Rosemond, Dr. Justin Stein and Mr. Joseph Silber to serve as representatives of the Society on an Action and Planning Committee on Breast Cancer Control. The Survey Committee placed great emphasis on the word "Action."

The Action and Planning Committee on Breast Cancer Control was appointed and met in New York City on Sunday, October 10, 1971. Committee members included:

Benjamin F. Byrd, Jr., M.D.
S. G. Cicetti
Gerald D. Dodd, M.D.
Robert V. P. Hutter, M.D.
Floyd Roos, M.D.
George P. Rosemond, M.D.

Joseph S. Silber
Ruth Snyder, M.D.
Justin J. Stein, M.D.
Phillip Strax, M.D.
Herman C. Zuckerman, M.D.

It was charged with the following responsibilities:

1. Review the current status of breast cancer control and the effectiveness of diagnostic modalities now in use.
2. Review programs for early detection of breast cancer now in progress.
3. Discuss problems of equipment, cost, personnel training, and mechanism for implementing programs which would hopefully save more lives from breast cancer.
4. Recommend approaches for adoption and implementation by the National Society and its Divisions.

The discussion provided the expert opinions of radiologists, surgeons, pathologists, a senior lay volunteer and a Division Executive Vice President. A parallel was drawn between the early days of the Pap Smear program of the Society and the subsequent striking reduction in the mortality from cancer of the cervix. It was pointed out that the American College of Radiology has some on-going mammography programs, funded federally, and that most of these programs were investigative rather than service oriented. The limitations and advantages of clinical examination, mammography and thermography were reviewed in detail, as were the cost factors of breast cancer detection programs. The newer pathologic concept of "minimal breast cancer" was described and the program of the New York City Division which includes a mobile unit was defined.

The Committee unanimously approved the following resolution for referral to a special session of the Medical and Scientific Executive Committee.

WHEREAS, it is agreed that the mortality rate of breast cancer has not changed significantly in the past 35 years, and

WHEREAS, the hope for immediate improvement in the results of breast cancer treatment lies in *earlier* diagnosis, be it therefore

RESOLVED: that the American Cancer Society develop and implement a major program designed to diagnose breast cancer at the earliest possible stage, and to obtain this goal the following recommendations are made:

1. That earlier diagnosis of breast cancer can now be achieved by a combination of clinical examination, mammography and thermography along with expanded Public Education programs for breast self-examination and Profes-

sional Education programs which alert physicians to the importance of breast cancer control and provide information about how best to perform adequate breast examinations.

2. That cooperation be sought from federal agencies, professional organizations and organized medical societies to enlarge the scope of the program.

3. That programs of training of radiologists and their personnel be developed and supported financially as soon as possible to provide the skills and staff needed to render competent service to the American public.

4. That the prototype mobile unit designed for reaching women in outlying communities be developed in several large cities through the sponsorship of appropriate and interested Divisions.

5. That a professional film be prepared as soon as possible and when funds are available for the purpose of informing the profession about the principles of a sound program for the earlier detection of breast cancer and that this film be distributed widely to medical schools, hospitals, professional organizations, medical societies, etc.

6. That the Public Education Committee continue to list a "lump in the breast" as a warning signal of cancer, although it is recognized that the lump which is cancer could possibly have been so diagnosed before it was palpable.

7. That serious consideration be given to supporting large centers which already have the equipment and staff to conduct programs of earlier detection of breast cancer, and that support be provided for screening programs which include the detection of uterine cancer simultaneously.

8. That adequate funds be made available in the research and clinical investigation programs of the Society to support physicians and scientists who are studying special aspects of mammography, thermography and other diagnostic modalities designed to detect early breast cancer.

In summary, the Action and Planning Committee on Breast Cancer recommends that the American Cancer Society assume a prominent and historic leadership role in bringing to the public those facilities and talents which are needed to reduce the excessive mortality from breast cancer. The Committee expressed a sense of urgency about launching a massive attack on the breast cancer problem and the Committee was of the opinion that there were enough new developments in diagnostic techniques and pathologic concepts to do so very soon. The Medical and Scientific Executive Committee is being asked to evaluate these recommendations and lead the way to a proper beginning.

The Medical and Scientific Executive Committee enthusiastically endorsed these recommendations in principle for long-term planning and felt that a mechanism is needed to develop specific programs which could be initiated as soon as possible.

The Medical and Scientific Executive Committee recommends that the American Cancer Society accept as a firm and urgent commitment the essential steps toward the better control of breast cancer and that a Special Task Force on Breast Cancer be appointed to study, organize and develop these programs which will improve the present capacity for the earlier diagnosis of breast cancer and result in a significant reduction in mortality.

November 1971

Appendix II

September 18, 1972

Dr. Nathaniel I. Berlin
National Cancer Institute
Bethesda, Maryland 20014

Dear Nat:

I enjoyed meeting with you and Art last week and I think we made a great deal of progress. In the following I have tried to summarize the tentative agreements we reached:

1. Specifics Concerning Breast Cancer Demonstration Projects

a) Dr. Berlin would provide a protocol which can be sent to applicants.
b) Protocol would not require double blind studies.
c) Although not required, independent readings of test results would be desirable.
d) Protocol would require approval of hospital ethics committee or its equivalent.

2. ACS study groups would become combined ACS-NCI study groups with the addition of a pathologist and biometrician to each of the existing study groups. These additions to be chosen by NCI. Tentative appointees are as follows:

Pathologists:	Hutter	Zippin
	Hartman	Levin
	Gallagher	Taylor
		Dunn

3. Combined study groups would perform site visits (which NCI requires) as part of the reviewing process. The cost of site visits will be funded by NCI.

4. Combined study groups make recommendations to the ACS-NCI DIAGNOSTIC CONTROL ACTIVITIES GROUP. This group of 16, half from ACS and half from NCI, would have a co-chairman from each organization. The group would include radiologists, surgeons, internists and others such as epidemiologists to serve as reviewing group for all combined diagnostic control activities.

5. Applications approved by the DIAGNOSTIC CONTROL ACTIVITIES GROUP will then be routed concurrently to the Service and Rehabilitation

Committee of the ACS and to the appropriate reviewing body of the NCI. Funding, preferably on a fixed percentage basis, will then be directly from ACS and NCI to the applicant facility.

6. Processing of 8 ACS Breast Cancer Detection Projects now in hand.

The grant applications are now being reviewed by the ACS study groups. Each applicant will be contacted and offered the option of having his application considered for the combined program with the advantages of the combined program explained.

Those that prefer to remain with ACS will, if approved by the ACS study group, be referred to the National Service and Rehabilitation Committee and on to the Board for funding action.

Those that opt for the combined program will be further reviewed by the NCI appointees to the study groups and will have a site visit by the study group. These applicants will receive a revised protocol and will be asked to submit a supplemental or revised budget. The applications will then be processed by the National Service and Rehabilitation Committee of the ACS and by the appropriate NCI reviewing body and funding will be directly from ACS and NCI to the grantee.

It is estimated that this additional reviewing can be accomplished by the end of the year (1972).

7. ACS will provide for NCI before October 16:

lists of facilities preparing grant applications including address and name of facility and name of project director

budget analysis of 8 ACS projects in hand, including breakdown of personnel by type and patient fee estimated

8. NCI will provide for ACS:

Breast Cancer Demonstration Project protocol (see 1.a.)
extracts of HIP and Jefferson protocols
data sheets
statistical procedures

9. Periodic meetings, probably twice a year, of the principal investigators of all participating projects will be planned and budgeted for.

You mentioned that you were going to go through this same process and I look forward to your comments and suggestions.

Sincerely yours,

William M. Markel, M.D.

WMM:et
bcc: Reader File

DEPARTMENT OF HEALTH, EDUCATION, AND WELFARE
PUBLIC HEALTH SERVICE
NATIONAL INSTITUTES OF HEALTH
BETHESDA, MARYLAND 20014

18 September 1972

Dr. Arthur I. Holleb
Dr. William Markell
American Cancer Society
219 E. 42nd Street
New York, New York   10017

Dear Art and Bill:

I want to take this opportunity to do two things. One is to thank you very much for everything you did for me while I was in New York. While I cannot recall specifically thanking you for that magnificent lunch, I want to do so and do so appropriately.

I enjoyed very much the opportunity of meeting with you and with Dick Magrail to take the necessary steps to implement our desire to join with you in the support of the Breast Cancer Detection Units. I would like to take this opportunity also to let you know what I consider to be some of the issues that were raised and resolved. I have on a separate page outlined the review mechanism of the American Cancer Society. We have agreed that proposals could be submitted to the National Cancer Institute some place around Step 5 or 6 of the attached table. We have also agreed that you would add to your study group a pathologist and an epidemiologist. We have suggested the names of Drs. Hutter, Hartmann, and Gallagher for pathology and Drs. Taylor, Levin, Zippin, and Dunn in biometry. I have agreed that these groups could and should serve also as the project site visitors for the NCI and that the NCI would pay for the cost of the project site visits since that is a requirement that we make and you do not make.

I have also suggested that we add to our present Ad Hoc Diagnostic Control Committee, whose membership is attached, an approximately equal number of members to be nominated by the American Cancer Society. I look forward with great pleasure to receiving these names from you, and I will then proceed within the Institute to add them to the committee. At the same time you have agreed that you would consider within the American Cancer Society having this constitute the American Cancer Society's Diagnostic Control Advisory Committee.

I have agreed to review the need for an Ethics Committee Review by each one of the projects.

I have agreed to supply you a modified HIP and Jefferson protocol for the American Cancer Society. Incidentally, I worked on that on the plane coming home and the girls are now in the process of typing a draft. I do not anticipate that I will finish that before I leave but will send it to you shortly after I return home.

The National Cancer Institute will select an investigator and institution to manage the central coordinating office. We have suggested the names of Dr. Edmond Gehan at M.D. Anderson; Dr. Christopher Klimt, University of Maryland; Dr. Calvin Zippin, University of California; Dr. Charles MacMahan, Louisiana State University; and Dr. Cutler has suggested Dr. Zimmerman, and after meeting with you I thought I might add Dr. Marvin Zelen at the State University of New York at Buffalo. I am beginning to call some of these people to determine whether or not they would be interested.

I am hoping to get from you some analysis of where your projects will be located geographically. At the same time we also hope to have some analysis by your office of the various budgets. Parenthetically, I did look at a number of the budgets on my way home and find that I do not believe it should be too difficult to set up a table comparing the budget from each of the institutions.

This presents most of the things we agreed upon but should not be held to constitute a set of minutes. Needless to say, I believe that we have come a long way in exploring all the facets of the review and approval mechanisms of both the American Cancer Society and the National Cancer Institute. I am quite confident that at our next meeting we should be able to come to have drafts of a working document specifying each of the procedures to be carried out.

Very sincerely yours,

Nathaniel I. Berlin, M.D.
Director, Division of Cancer
Biology and Diagnosis
National Cancer Institute

Attachments
cc: Dr. Markell

Appendix III

Name and Mailing Address	*Project Director*
Breast Cancer Demonstration Project Department of Radiology Arizona Medical Center Tucson, Arizona 85724	Dr. Arthur J. Present
Breast Cancer Detection Center University of Southern California Room 7350A 1200 North State Street Los Angeles, California 90033	Dr. Lewis W. Guiss

Breast Screening Clinic of N. Calif. Dr. Robert Schweitzer
Samuel Merritt Hospital
384 34th Street
Oakland, California 94609

Breast Cancer Demonstration Project Dr. Bruce Schnider
Georgetown Hospital Dr. John Potter
Department of Neurology
3800 Resevoir Road
Washington, D.C. 20007

Breast Cancer Demonstration Project Dr. Leslie W. Whitney
Wilmington General Division
2nd North Area
Chestnut and Broom Streets
Wilmington, Delaware 19805

Breast Cancer Detection Center Dr. Marvin V. McClow
c/o St. Vincent's Medical Center
Barrs Street & St. Johns Ave.
Jacksonville, Florida 32203

Breast Cancer Demonstration Project Dr. Robert L. Brown
Emory University Dr. Robert L. Egan
Atlanta, Georgia 30322

Breast Screening Project Dr. A. Hamblin Letton
Georgia Baptist Hospital
340 Boulevard N.E., Suite 516
Atlanta, Georgia 30312

Breast Cancer Demonstration Center Dr. Fred I. Gilbert, Jr.
Pacific Health Research Institute
Alexander Young Building, Suite 545
Hotel & Bishop Streets
Honolulu, Hawaii 96813

Breast Cancer Detection Center Dr. Elisabeth Ward
Mountain States Tumor Institute
215 Avenue B
Boise, Idaho 83702

Breast Cancer Demonstration Project Dr. Donald C. Young
Iowa Lutheran Hospital
University and Penn Streets
Des Moines, Iowa 50316

Breast Cancer Demonstration Project Dr. Loren J. Humphrey—Director
University of Kansas Medical Center Dr. Robert Boudet—Project
Rainbow Boulevard at 39th Street   Coordinator
Kansas City, Kansas 66103

Breast Cancer Demonstration Project   Dr. Condict Moore
University of Louisville School of
    Medicine
627 Floyd Street
Louisville, Kentucky 40201

Breast Cancer Demonstration Project   Dr. Barbara Threatt
University Hospital
Dept. of Radiology
Room S-4432
1405 E. Ann. St.
Ann Arbor, Michigan 48104

Breast Cancer Demonstration Project   Dr. Ned Rodes
Ellis Fischel State Cancer Hospital
Business Loop—70th and Garth Ave.
Columbia, Missouri 65201

Breast Cancer Demonstration Project   Dr. Benjamin Rush
College of Medicine and Dentistry of
    New Jersey
100 Bergen Street
Newark, New Jersey 07103

Breast Cancer Demonstration Project   Dr. Philip Strax
Guttman Institute
200 Madison Avenue
New York, New York 10013

Breast Cancer Demonstration Project   Dr. Robert McClellan
Duke University Medical Center
Durham, North Carolina 27710

Breast Cancer Detection Center   Dr. Myron Moskowitz
University of Cincinnati Med. Ctr.
Logan Hall Basement, Room 10E
Cincinnati, Ohio 45229

Breast Cancer Screening Center   Dr. JoAnn D. Haberman
Oklahoma Medical Research
    Foundation Building
825 N.E. 13th Street
Oklahoma City, Oklahoma 73190

Breast Cancer Demonstration Project   Dr. Morton J. Goodman
Good Samaritan Hospital and Medical
    Center
2222 N.W. Lovejoy
Portland, Oregon 97210

Breast Cancer Demonstration Project Albert Einstein Medical Center York and Tabor Roads Philadelphia, Pennsylvania 19141	Dr. Harold J. Isard
Breast Cancer Demonstration Project Temple University Hospital 3401 North Broad Street Philadelphia, Pennsylvania 19140	Dr. Marc S. Lapayowker
Statistical Center University City Science Center 3508 Science Center Philadelphia, Pennsylvania 19104	Dr. Perry Scheinok
Breast Cancer Demonstration Project University of Pittsburgh School of Medicine 3550 Terrace Street Pittsburgh, Pennsylvania 15261	Dr. Bernard Fisher
Breast Cancer Demonstration Project Rhode Island Hospital 593 Eddy Street—Room 141 Ambulatory Patient Center Providence, Rhode Island 02902	Dr. Herbert P. Constantine
Breast Cancer Demonstration Project Vanderbilt University Hospital Room 110, Baker Bldg. 110 21st Ave. South Nashville, Tennessee 37232	Dr. M. D. Ingram
Breast Cancer Detection Center St. Joseph's Hospital 707 St. Joseph's Professional Bldg. Houston, Texas 77002	Dr. Duncan L. Moore Dr. John E. Martin
Breast Cancer Demonstration Project Virginia Mason Clinic 1118 9th Ave. Seattle, Washington 98101	Dr. Thomas Carlile
Breast Cancer Demonstration Project Department of Radiology Medical College of Wisconsin 8700 W. Wisconsin Milwaukee, Wisconsin 53226	Dr. John Milbrath Dr. James E. Youker—Co-Director

Appendix IV

DEPARTMENT OF HEALTH, EDUCATION, AND WELFARE
PUBLIC HEALTH SERVICE
NATIONAL INSTITUTES OF HEALTH
BETHESDA, MARYLAND 20014

National Cancer Institute

February 8, 1973

Saul Harris
Director, Office of Radiation Control
Department of Health—City of New York
325 Broadway
New York, New York 10007

Dear Mr. Harris:

In reply to your letter of January 10, 1973 to Dr. Frank J. Rauscher, Jr., Director of the National Cancer Institute, concerning the proposed and almost operational American Cancer Society and National Cancer Institute Breast Cancer Demonstration Projects, I would like to indicate that there have been several meetings of competent radiologists who have the opinion of several physicists that mammography, as it is done now in centers with competent personnel, has relatively little risk of causing excessive x-ray exposure to the patients so examined.

Techniques vary from one institute to another, but none of the techniques that are regularly employed will give more than seven to eight rads per breast for each examination. It is quite difficult to establish what is the carcinogenic dose for breast cancer, but it is generally agreed to be quite high. Except possibly in very special instances where mass exposure has been given, as in Hiroshima, there is no real evidence that x-ray has produced mammary cancer. Mammography, as used in this country, has not produced breast cancer to our knowledge.

I am enclosing the opinion of one of our consultants in mammography and he indicates what the dose is at his particular institution and some data on other methods used. Most radiologists are studying methods to reduce the radiation dose and there are techniques available which will probably prove to be quite satisfactory that give a dose of only 1–1.5 rads per exposure. These examinations will be given to women over 35 and the vast majority will be beyond the child bearing age and hence, genetic dangers will not be a great factor.

It is evident to all of us that the least exposure to x-irradiation is desirable. Breast cancer is a real danger and a cause of death in approximately 30,000 women a year in this country. This high mortality makes the remote danger of x-ray causing cancer a permissible and calculated risk.

I think the National Cancer Institute through its consulting committees have explored all of the possible dangers of mammography and feel that its benefits far outweigh any potential dangers.

Thank you for your inquiry and if you have further questions, please feel free to communicate with us.

Sincerely yours,

(Signed)
Kenneth B. Olson, M.D.
Diagnosis Program Officer
Division of Cancer Biology
 and Diagnosis
National Cancer Institute

Enclosure
CC: Dr. Dodd
    Dr. Lester
    Dr. Strax

8. References

1. National Cancer Institute, Cancer Patient Survival Report No. 5, 1976, DHEW Publication No. (NIH)77–992, National Cancer Institute, Bethesda, Maryland (1977).
2. *American Cancer Society Facts and Figures 1980*, American Cancer Society, New York (1979).
3. L. Heuser, J. S. Spratt, Jr., H. C. Polk, Jr., and J. Buchanan, Relation between mammary cancer growth kinetics and the intervals between screenings, *Cancer* 43, 857–862 (1979).
4. M. L. Levin and D. B. Thomas, Epidemiology of breast cancer, in: *Progress in Clinical and Biological Research*, Vol. 12 (A. C. W. Montague *et al.*, eds.), pp. 9–35, Alan R. Liss, New York (1977).
5. Final Reports of National Cancer Institute Ad Hoc Groups on Mammography Screening for Breast Cancer and a Summary Report of Their Joint Findings and Recommendations, DHEW Publication No. (NIH) 77–1400, National Cancer Institute, Bethesda, Maryland (March 1977).
6. A. I. Holleb, Magnitude of the breast cancer problem in the United States, in: *Progress in Clinical and Biological Research*, Vol. 12 (A. C. W. Montague *et al.*, eds.), pp. 3–7, Alan R. Liss, New York (1977).
7. American Cancer Society, Circular Letter, MA-15, New York, February 23 (1972).
8. National Cancer Institute, Report of the Working Group to Review the NCI/ACS Breast Cancer Demonstration Detection Projects (NCI Contract No. RFP-NO1-CN-75379), (September 1977).
9. D. H. McGregor, C. E. Land, K. Choi, S. Tokuoka, P. Liu, T. Wakabayashi, and G. W. Beebe, Breast cancer incidence among atomic bomb survivors of Hiroshima and Nagasaki 1950–69, Atomic Bomb Casualty Commission, Japanese National Institute of

Health of the Ministry of Health and Welfare, Technical Report 32–71. Revised 22 August 1975.

10. J. C. Bailar III, Mammographic screening: A reappraisal of benefits and risks, *Clin. Obstet. Gynecol.* **21**, 1–14 (1978).

11. B. F. Byrd, Jr., ACS/NCI breast cancer detection demonstration projects, *Cancer* **46**, 1084–1086 (1980).

12. L. S. Brinton, R. R. Williams, R. N. Hoover, N. L. Stegens, M. Seinleib, and J. F. Fraumeni, Jr., Breast cancer risk factors among screening program participants, *J. Natl. Cancer Inst.* **62**, 37–44 (1979).

13. Report of the Subcommittee on Follow-up of the Breast Cancer Detection Demonstration Project, L. H. Baker and G. Metter, chairmen, September 8 (1978) (unpublished).

14. W. H. Hartmann, The pathology of the ACS/NCI Breast Cancer Detection Demonstration Projects—a status report, Given at the American Cancer Society's National Conference—breast cancer, New York (1979).

6

Reconstruction of the Female Breast after Mastectomy

REUVEN K. SNYDERMAN

1. Introduction

Reconstruction of the female breast after mastectomy has been carried out for many years. The early cases were done shortly after the World War I, when plastic surgery in the United States had a major surge of growth. Over the years, the procedures that were used for reconstructing the breast were complicated. Normally, a number of surgical operations were necessary. The patient had to be returned to the hospital frequently, and the time to complete the surgery was long. Many reconstructions took as long as a year or a year and a half. The total length of time was increased by minor or major complications. It could well be said that by the time the reconstruction was completed, the surgeon was tired of the patient and patient was tired of the surgeon. Because of this, few reconstructions were carried out. However, the literature shows individual cases in which plastic surgeons were indeed innovative in carrying out a suitable manner of reconstruction. One of the major defects, however, in reconstructing the breast was the scars created in other areas as flaps and tube pedicles were formed and moved into position.

The modern era of breast reconstruction started about ten years ago. This basically was brought about by three factors:

1. The development of the silicone prosthesis. The silicone prosthesis has been used for augmentation mammoplasties for about

REUVEN K. SNYDERMAN • College of Medicine/Dentistry of New Jersey–Rutgers Medical School, University Heights, Piscataway, New Jersey 08854.

20 years. Constant improvement finally gave us a very useful
and workable prosthesis.

2. Approximately ten years ago, a lesser operation for treatment of
   carcinoma of the breast began to be used more often. This is the
   modified radical mastectomy in which the pectoralis muscles are
   left behind. This leaves a woman who is more suitable for reconstruction and who can be reconstructed in an easier manner.

3. The women's liberation movement and other such groups
   brought about a demand that they take a more active part in
   deciding the type of surgery that would be carried out on them.
   Many women would insist when a suspicious lump was found
   that the biopsy be done and the patient then be awakened and
   allowed to discuss the future surgery with her surgeon. Before
   that time, it was quite common to admit the patient to the hospital, have a biopsy and a frozen section, and if this proved to be
   cancer, perform the mastectomy at the same operation.

In addition, as reconstruction was publicized, the women's groups
themselves demanded information from their ablative surgeons and
women's magazines began to feature articles describing reconstruction.

There are approximately 90,000 mastectomies per year being performed in the United States. It is our belief that about 80% of these
women are able to readjust after the surgery to their premastectomy
state. This means that they are able to return to their homes and to live
satisfactory lives with their husbands and children. About 20% are
probably unable to adjust, and these women should be given the opportunity of discussing reconstructive surgery with a plastic surgeon who is
interested in the subject. A simple referral to any plastic surgeon is not
satisfactory, for if he is not interested in the problem, he may discourage
the woman from seeking further help. Approximately ten years ago, one
of five patients coming in for consultation for reconstruction underwent
the surgery. Today, about three of five patients who come in for consultation are undergoing reconstructive surgery.

Reconstructive surgery is not the first thing that should be offered to
the woman who has had a mastectomy and who is having problems. It is
important that she be given the chance to discuss her problem with her
ablative surgeon. Frequently, the patient is unaware of the meaning of
the tightness in the chest wall and what the swelling of the arm indicates, and deep down believes that these are signs of further cancer. She
should also have had the opportunity of being fitted properly for an
external prosthesis. This means more than just sending her to a local
lingerie shop with a note. The prosthesis should be fitted and then
checked by the ablative surgeon or his representative to make sure that
the woman really has obtained the best prosthesis available.

Some women need to be referred for physical therapy to help loosen the chest wall and upper extremity. Agencies such as Reach to Recovery and Encore have done much along these lines to help the woman. Where marital problems existed before the surgery, they can only become more acute afterward. It is necessary to discuss the problem of the mastectomy not only with the patient but also with her husband or male partner. If the problem is more severe than the ablative surgeon can handle, then the use of psychiatric help should be considered.

It is only after all these modalities have been exhausted that the patient should be referred for reconstructive surgery.

Today, however, it is not uncommon for the ablative surgeon to discuss with his patient the possibility of reconstruction even before she has the mastectomy. On occasion, the reconstructive surgeon may even be asked to see the patient premastectomy to discuss with her what can be done for her in the future. Many a tearful patient, the night before her mastectomy, has been relieved by a brief discussion and assurance that in the future reconstructive surgery is possible for her.

2. Initial Interview

The initial interview must be a lengthy one. My own routine is to see the patient alone, even if she has come with her spouse. After carrying out an examination, I question her in detail concerning what she knows about the surgery that has been performed. It is interesting to find out what she has been told about the type of surgery and about the findings of her lymph nodes. She is questioned as to whether she is on chemotherapy or has had any radiation therapy. A breast history of her family, to see which members may have had carcinoma, is also of aid. It is important to obtain from the ablative surgeon a copy of the surgical procedure and his pathology findings. Frequently, women bring this with them to the initial interview. It is repeated over and over to the woman that reconstruction can be carried out but that a cosmetic triumph will not be obtained. It is important to make sure that the woman understands this, for not only do some patients feel that they will look as good after reconstructive surgery, but also some actually feel they will look even better.

It is important at the initial interview to find out exactly what the problem is for the patient. It is sometimes difficult to evaluate this. Some will state that they are unable to find a prosthesis that fits, or that, being athletic, they find that the prosthesis moves out when they are pursuing the sport. Others may complain only of a scar that is unsightly and limits the type of clothes that they can wear. The methods of reconstruction are then discussed with the patient and photographs of pre- and post-operative appearance are shown. The patient is discouraged at that point of making a decision, and once again she is told to realize that the reconstruction will not be a cosmetic triumph. Jokingly, I tell them that they will not be a candidate for the centerfold of *Playboy* magazine. The husband or male partner is brought into the room, and in front of the patient I usually assure the wife that the husband will support her whether or not she has the reconstruction. The husband is usually anxious to agree with this, for if the husband is pushing for the reconstruction, then there is usually a marital problem that is not going to be improved or solved by the breast reconstruction. On completion of the interview, we offer the patient a chance to speak with other women who have undergone reconstruction. We have a list of patients who are more than willing to do this, and we try to match up the patient with someone in her age group. Frequently, the patient will have made up her mind by the end of the first interview that this is what she desires. Others will have been turned off completely, stating that the photographs that they saw are not acceptable to them and they do not feel that what can be given to them would be of any benefit to their own self-image. Either direction the patient chooses to go is fine. Some choose to give it some thought and return for a second interview and further discussion.

It is interesting to note that some women, after looking at the photographs and listening to discussion, will turn and ask "Do you do facelifts?" as they move their hands over their faces and push the skin around. These women are basically looking for some type of surgical procedure to give them a lift at an emotionally low point in their life. If the discussion goes in this direction, I am more than pleased to discuss the possibility with them, and we have carried out facelift procedures on a number of patients who had mastectomies who choose never to have breast reconstruction.

The woman who has undergone a mastectomy complains of the following problems: (1) lack of a mound; (2) subclavicular defects; (3) an axillary hollow; and (4) scars. The alternatives that are available to correct these defects today are discussed in the following section.

3. Alternative Types of Reconstruction Today

3.1. Revision of a Scar

As stated before, some of the patients in their initial interview will state that what is really bothering them is the fact that a scar protrudes beyond a certain type of garment that they wish to wear. If this is the patient's main complaint, a discussion should be only in the direction of what can be done to improve the scar. A patient with a dog-ear left from the original mastectomy can have it repaired and flattened to give the patient the result that she wants.

3.2. Reduction of the Remaining Breast (Fig. 1)

Women who have large breasts and have a mastectomy are left with a large remaining breast that frequently they cannot match with a stan-

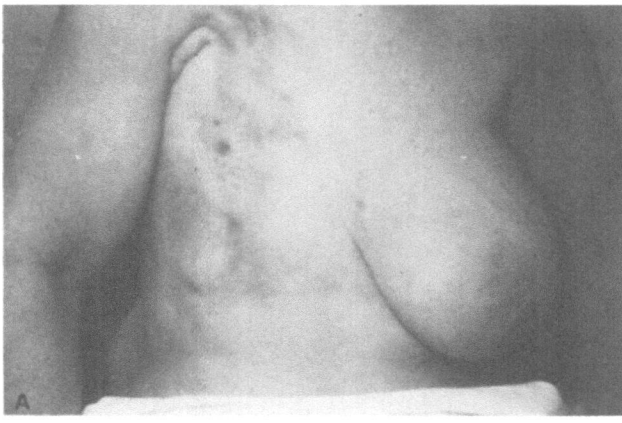

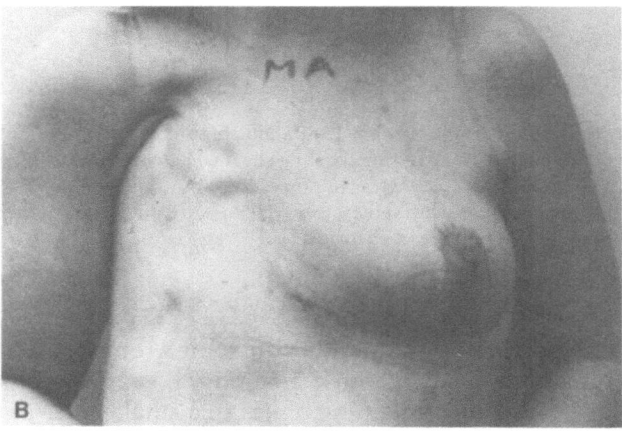

Fig. 1. (A) After radical mastectomy with remaining breast large and possibly hypertrophy since surgery. (B) Following elevation–reduction mammoplasty by a standard Strombeck method. The patient is now able to wear a smaller external prosthesis and finds it easier to match the remaining breast.

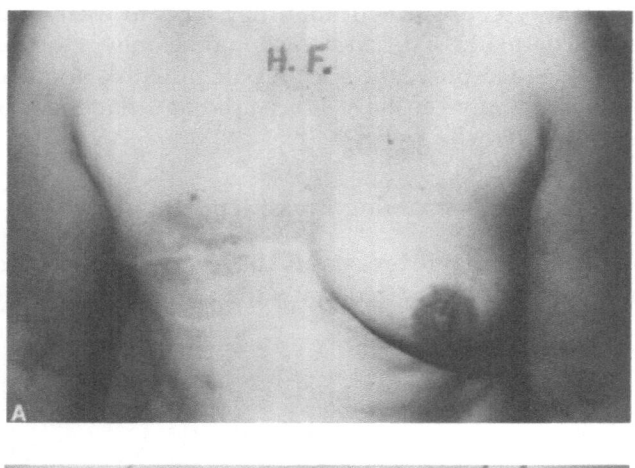

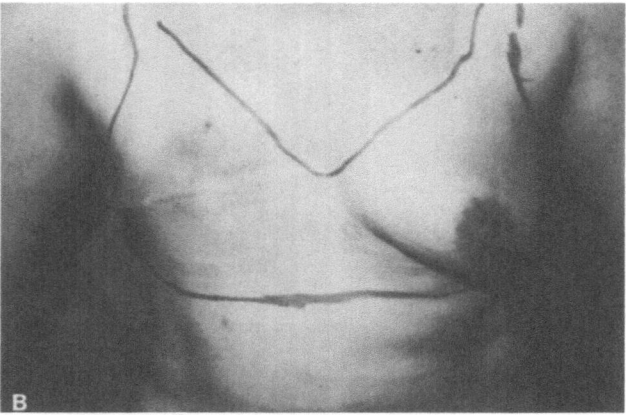

Fig. 2. (A) After modified mastectomy. (B) Patient brought to the operating room with the bra in position, which is then outlined on the chest wall to help locate the position of the prosthesis. (C) Postoperative view showing insertion of the silicone prosthesis only. The volume and shape of the breast are satisfactory. (D) Postoperative view in the bra, showing breast equality and the presence of cleavage.

dard external prosthesis. In addition, in some women, after a mastectomy, the remaining breast will hypertrophy. For these women, reduction and elevation of the remaining breast to a smaller size and different shape will make it easier for them to obtain an external prosthesis. Some women desire only this and are pleased with the final results and are able to continue wearing external prostheses in their bras.

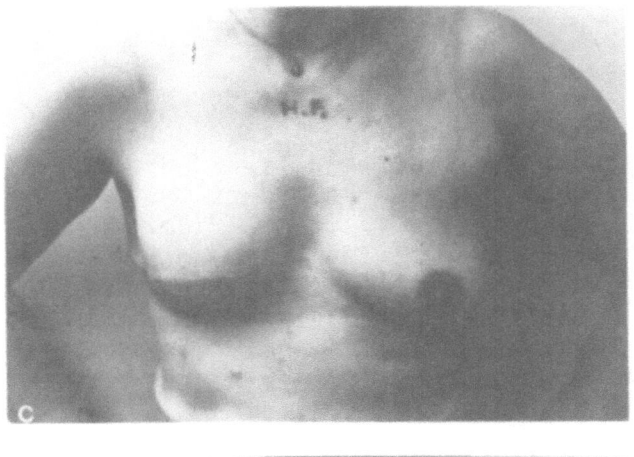

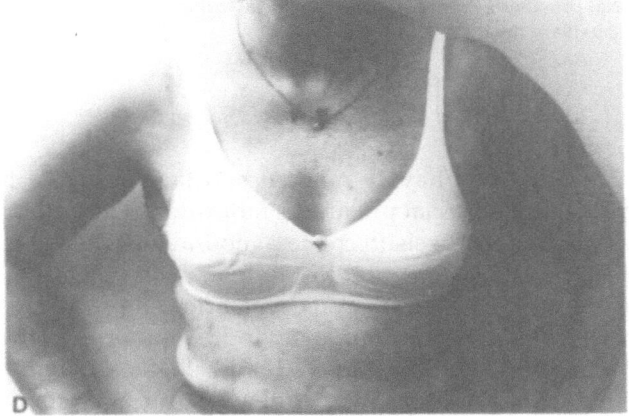

Fig. 2 (*cont.*)

3.3. Insertion of the Prosthesis Only (Fig. 2)

To the woman who has had a modified mastectomy and has a remaining small breast, reconstruction can be simply carried out by the insertion of a prosthesis alone. Total operating time might be an hour or less. The silicone prosthesis can be placed in a pocket created in the mastectomy side, and the size can approach that of the remaining breast. If she desires, an areolar nipple complex can be made at a later time.

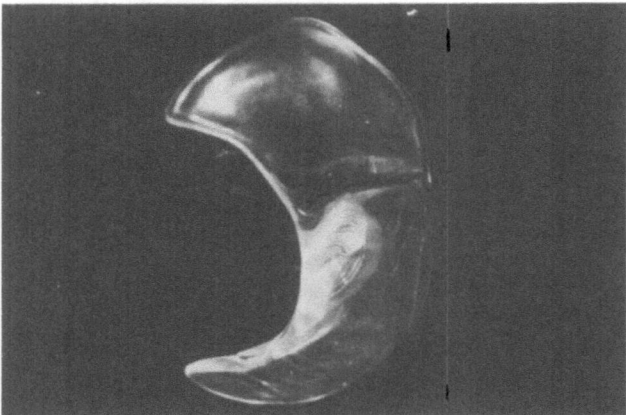

Fig. 3. A special prosthesis fabricated to fill a subclavicular defect. The prosthesis may be inserted to the axillary area.

3.4. Use of a Special Prosthesis (Fig. 3)

Some patients who have a marked subclavicular defect can have this filled by having a special prosthesis fabricated. The patient may first have had a regular prosthesis to create a mound and then at a later time have a special prosthesis inserted through an axillary incision to fill the subclavicular defect. Or, one specially prefabricated prosthesis may both fill the subclavicular area and form a mound. A moulage of the patient's chest is made and refined to the size and shape desired. It is then fabricated by one of the prosthesis companies out of silicone. They are able to fill it either with liquid silicone or, if it is desired to give a firmer edge to the prosthesis, with a firmer type of silicone. This prosthesis can then be inserted in one operation and give a quite acceptable result.

3.5. Reconstruction of the Areolar Nipple Complex

It is interesting to note that many women coming in for consultation will ask immediately how an areolar nipple would be formed. We assure them that we can do this, perhaps briefly tell them of the methods, and then pass on to further discussion. However, the patients will continue to return to the subject over and over again. Actually, when the woman has a mound created, and no areolar nipple complex is made at that time, many of them will forget that they ever were concerned about the areolar nipple complex and will not have it formed at all.

An areolar nipple complex can be made by saving the areolar tissue removed from the other breast if it needs to be elevated and reduced. It can also be made of a portion of the labia. However, this tends to lead to a painful scar, and I have abandoned that method of reconstruction. Probably the easiest method is to take a circle of darkened skin from the upper, inner thigh. At a later date, either a nipplelike complex can be made by advancing the center of the areola by simple V–Y incision or a small graft can be inserted from the lobule of the ear or a portion of the toe.

Some patients will be satisfied with the use of dye, such as lipstick, and others have had an areola tattooed on the reconstructed chest wall.

3.6. Combination of These Methods (Figs. 4 and 5)

The one-stage surgical procedure, as I choose to call it, for reconstruction of the female breast after mastectomy today is an operation of about 2½ hr in duration. The patient may be hospitalized for 2 or 3 days, but leaves the hospital in a bra and markedly improved emotionally.

The patient is brought to the operating room in a bra and a prosthesis to which she has become accustomed. On her chest wall, the bra is outlined with a marking pen. On the mastectomy side, a line 4–6 cm long is marked above the lower bra line. If the remaining breast is small, then nothing further need be marked. If it is large, it is marked for reduction. I personally make use of a Strombeck pattern. The patient's arms are taped to the abdomen in akimbo position. She is placed horizontally on the table, and under general anesthesia, the chest is prepped and draped. On the side to be reconstructed, the incision is made down to the chest wall, and all tissue, skin, subcutaneous tissue, fat, and any muscle fibers that are left are elevated. A pocket is created in the area where the breast should be. The outline of the bra on the chest wall helps to determine this. Sizer protheses are kept sterile in the operating room, and these are tried until the desired prosthesis size is obtained. One must not overstuff the pocket, for if one does so, the overlying tissue may well become necrotic. Also, if one puts in too large a prosthesis, the chance that a scar capsule will form is greater. A few simple sutures will close the wound over the temporary prosthesis.

The remaining breast is then treated like any other elevation and reduction. The areolar nipple complex is marked to reduce it in size. The extra areolar tissue is removed and saved until the end of the operation. The keyhole flap is then denuded of the epithelium, the breast is reduced as necessary, and key sutures are placed. The patient is then placed in a sitting position, and the two breasts are checked for size, volume, and shape. Further reduction can be carried out if necessary. The elevated and reduced breast is then checked for hemastasis. A drain

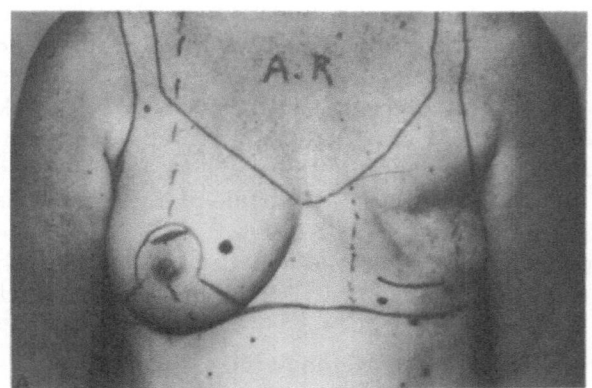

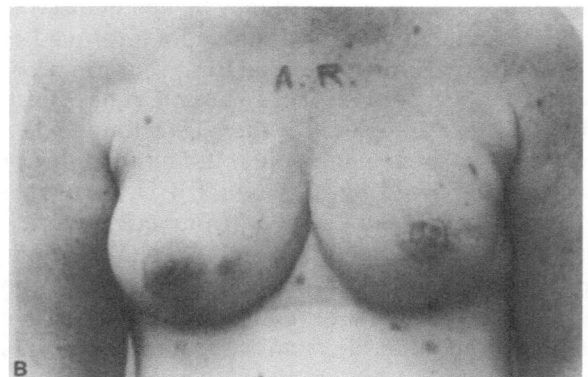

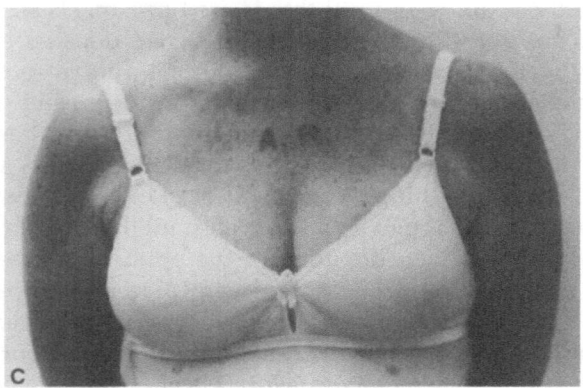

may or may not be used, and the wound is closed in the usual manner making use of fine silk, nylon, and subcutaneous sutures of catgut.

On the reconstructed side, the sizer prosthesis is removed, and a sterile prosthesis of the same size is then inserted. Before this is done, hemastasis is checked and the pocket is syringed out. All wounds are then closed. The patient is again placed in the sitting position, and only now is the location for the new areolar nipple complex marked. There appears to be no way that this can be done preoperatively, since the shape of the reconstructed breast will probably not be the same as the elevated–reduced one, and while measurements may help, it is basically a visual inspection that allows for the proper placement of the areolar complex. The patient is then returned to the recumbent position. The superficial epithelium is removed from the newly marked nipple area. The areolar tissue that was saved from the other side is then sutured into position. If there is little tissue, it can be twisted around in a ciruclar manner and stretched. One may even bunch a little bit up in the center to simulate a nipple. Xeroform, 2 × 2's, steri-strip dressing is applied, and a large wraparound dressing is placed on the patient. Forty-eight hours later, the drain is removed and the patient placed in a sleep bra—a bra with hooks in the front that holds the dressings in place. Providing there have been no problems, the patient may be discharged from the hospital in 3 days, the areolar dressing removed in about 7 days, and all sutures removed in about 2 weeks.

Possible complications, of course, include infection. We have had no real problem with this. Hematomas can develop, usually on the side that has the prosthesis. If it develops, the patient must have it evacuated, bleeding controlled, and a new prosthesis inserted. Only if the prosthesis is too large and the tension on the skin too great does the possibility of necrosis occur. Should this happen, there is no choice but to remove the implant, and further reconstruction will be necessary by means of a more complicated operation. Postoperatively, there are usually some shifts in the position of the reconstructed breast, and with time they may equalize.

The patient, of course, is told beforehand that the two breasts will not be perfectly equal, since few women have breasts that are equal.

Fig. 4. (A) Patient brought to the operating room with her bra outlined on her chest wall. The line of incision on the left side is marked for the creation of a pocket. The right breast is marked for elevation–reduction by a Strombeck pattern. (B) Postoperative view showing the right breast elevated and reduced. The left breast was reconstructed by silicone implants. An areolar nipple complex was formed out of tissue removed when elevating and reducing the right breast. (C) Postoperative view in the bra, showing the equal appearance of the breasts. There is good cleavage.

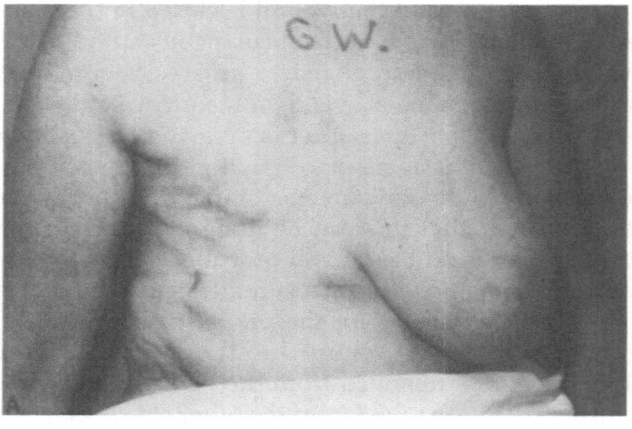

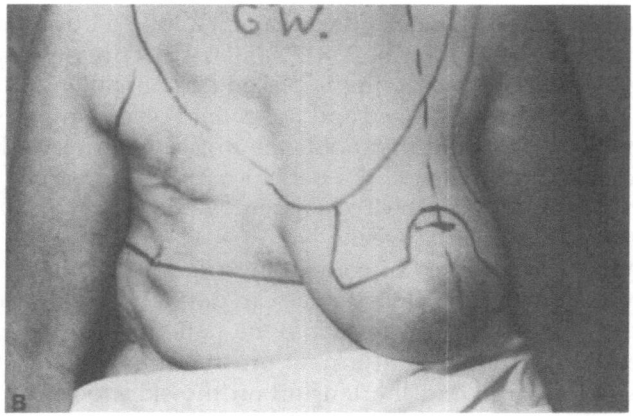

Fig. 5. (A) After right radical mastectomy with a large remaining breast. (B) The patient's bra is marked on the chest wall with the left breast marked for elevation and reduction. (C) Postoperative appearance showing the left breast elevated and reduced. The right breast was reconstructed by means of a silicone prosthesis. The areola was reconstructed from extra areolar tissue removed when elevating and reducing the left breast. (D) Postoperative view in the bra, showing equal-appearing breasts with fullness above the bra line.

The final photographs are always taken with a bra on. The patient is told over and over again that we hope to make her able to look well in a bra, tennis dress, or bikini. While she may look a great deal better in the nude than before the reconstruction, the goal of the operation is to make it possible for her to wear normal clothes.

The patient who complains of the inability to wear an external pros-

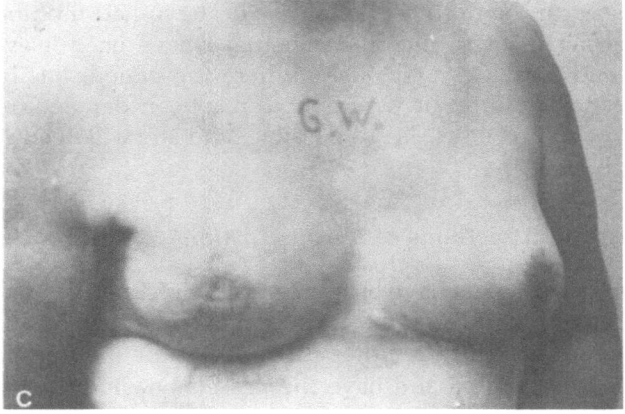

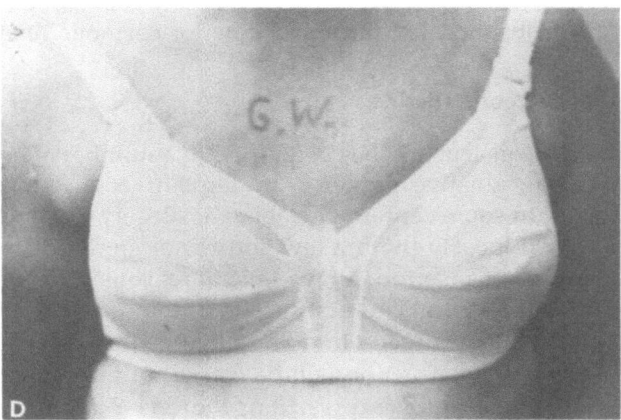

thesis is the one who is usually the most pleased with this surgery. Also, the ability to walk into a boutique and buy a normal bra without having to go through the embarrassment of being specially fitted produces a marked psychiatric improvement. Of the approximately 200 reconstructions that I have carried out in this manner, two patients were failures because of the extrusion of the prostheses. This was early on when I attempted to overstretch the pocket. The rest of the patients have all been pleased with the result of the surgery for the reason stated above.

A patient becomes eligible for this one-stage reconstruction approximately 6 months after the mastectomy wound is healed. This is possible when the tissue over the chest wall becomes freely movable. Basically, this operation can be used on patients who have had modified radical mastectomies. However, in some patients, I have used it even where they have had a radical. Obviously, where the patient has had a skin graft or extended radical or where there has been damage from radiation, this type of procedure is not possible, and she will need something more complicated.

3.7. Microsurgical Methods of Reconstruction

A number of centers have been attempting reconstruction by means of microvascular methods. Large areas of skin, subcutaneous tissue, and fat can be brought up from either the buttocks or the inguinal region directly to the chest area and have the vessels anastomosed to axillary vessels. At this time, this procedure does not seem to be a good one. Further investigation is necessary. The use of a myocutaneous flap (see Section 3.9) is probably safer and gives a better cosmetic result.

3.8. Immediate Reconstruction

Immediate reconstruction has been tried in a number of centers. On completion of the ablative surgery, an implant is inserted and the wound is closed. In some centers, the ablative surgery is completed, the wounds are closed loosely (with a few sutures or steri-strips), and in a few days an implant is inserted. I have several reasons for not endorsing this type of reconstruction. The first reason is that it might place some pressure on the ablative surgeon to do less than is necessary to obtain a cure knowing that reconstruction will be carried out immediately. Second, on the completion of the dissection, there is a large, raw surface that will tend, if not to bleed, at least to pour out serous fluid. When this happens, it is possible that the prosthesis will extrude either through the incision line or, if pressure is great enough, through any part of the flap. Third, the woman who had immediate reconstruction, and once again this also not being a cosmetic triumph, may well be disappointed in what she sees. The patient who has the opportunity of living 6 months or so in a postmastectomy state is far more appreciative of reconstruction.

3.9. Myocutaneous Flap (Fig. 6)

The development of the myocutaneous flap has now made it possible to reconstruct any woman who has had a mastectomy. Basically, the myocutaneous flap makes use of a muscle to transpose a paddle of skin. The muscle used for reconstruction of the breast is the latissimus dorsi.

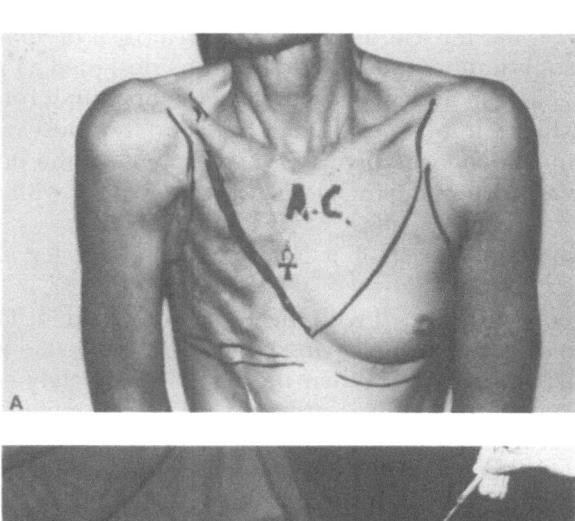

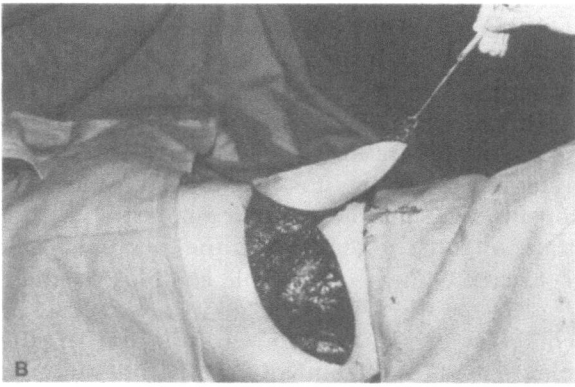

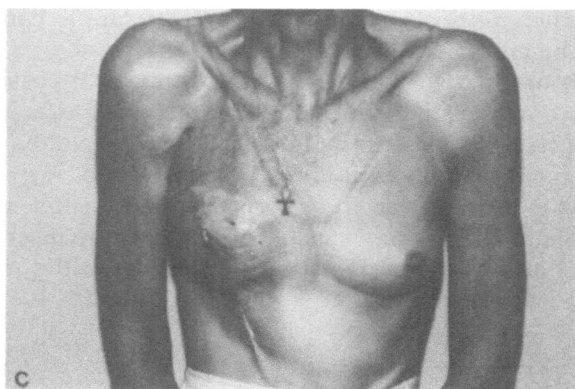

Fig. 6. (A) Preoperative view. The bra is marked and lines of incision are indicated. (B) Myocutaneous flap ready for rotation. (C) Postoperative view. The subclavicular defects are filled with muscle and the breast is reconstructed.

This is a large, flat muscle. It will give a great deal of volume, and the size of the superimposed skin paddle can be designed as needed.

Once again, the patient is brought to the operating room in her bra with the prothesis in place. This is outlined on the chest wall. The lines of incision for the myocutaneous flap are drawn on the posterior chest wall in such a way that the final line of closure will be within the normal bra line.

The remaining breast, if it is large, is marked for elevation and reduction.

The operation is started with the patient on her side. The latissimus dorsi is then dissected free, leaving connected to it a skin paddle of the desired length and width. When the flap is completely elevated, it is tunneled through in the axillary area and the posterior wound is closed.

The old scar on the mastectomy side is then excised, or if a skin graft is present, it is removed. The muscle is then sutured into position to give a subclavicular fill, and suturing is continued along the medial aspect toward the sternum. The silicone prosthesis is inserted behind the muscle, and the skin paddle is then fitted into position and the wounds are closed. If the remaining breast is small, no further work need be done. If the remaining breast is large, it is elevated and reduced to bring it into better relationship with the reconstructed breast.

The extra areolar tissue removed at the time of elevation–reduction is then used to create an areolar nipple complex on the reconstructed side.

If no work is necessary on the remaining breast, then no areolar nipple complex is made at the time of surgery, but rather a period of 3–6 months is allowed for the reconstructed side to soften and to shape itself, and then reconstruction of the areolar nipple complex can be carried out by any of the standard methods.

The use of the myocutaneous flap now makes it possible to reconstruct any woman despite the extent of surgery. If a skin graft has been used, it can be removed and replaced by the skin paddle. If tissue has been damaged by radiation, it may also be replaced.

When the tissue over the chest wall, no matter what type of surgery, has not become movable or loose enough to insert a prosthesis as described above by the one-stage method, then the myocutaneous flap becomes a necessity.

4. Chemotherapy

If a woman is undergoing chemotherapy, it is important to discuss with her chemotherapist the exact routine of her treatment. If she is to be receiving the therapy for only a year, then probably it would be best to wait until she completes the year. However, if the therapy is to run for a longer period of time and the woman is anxious to be reconstructed, there is no reason the reconstruction cannot be fitted into the chemotherapy regime. I personally will wait 3 or 4 weeks after the last treatment, carry out the reconstruction after having checked the patient's blood picture, and return her to her chemotherapist in time to carry on with little or no interruption of her chemotherapy routine.

5. Who Should Be Reconstructed?

There is no question that the patient who has the less malignant tumor and who has had lesser surgery is the ideal candidate for reconstruction. However, it is the woman herself who must make the final decision whether she wishes to have reconstruction. She should have had the chance of discussing her prognosis with her ablative surgeon. He should have discussed with her the type of tumor and probably such results as estrogen-receptor tests and other thoughts concerning her chance of survival for 5, 10, or 15 years. After being apprised of this information and after speaking with the reconstructive surgeon, the patient herself should be allowed to make the decision as to whether or not she wishes to have reconstruction. Basically, what we are talking about now is quality of life, and this must be the patient's own decision. Obviously, it is our responsibility to guide her in the right direction, but I do not think that we can close the door in her face and say, "No, you cannot be reconstructed because your tumor was malignant, your lymph nodes were positive, your estrogen-receptor test was negative, etc."

In my personal experience, I have had a patient who knew she had metastases but wished to have reconstruction. Fortunately, she needed only the simple insertion of a prosthesis, which was done in less than an hour. The patient's survival was only about 22 months, but at the last interview that I had with her, she stated that she was pleased that she had made the decision to be reconstructed.

6. Follow-up after Reconstructive Surgery

The patient should continue to be followed by her ablative surgeon as well as the plastic surgeon. Should there be recurrence, treatment would be the same as though she had not had reconstruction. X-ray therapy may be given through a prosthesis; however, the prosthesis can be easily removed and the X-ray therapy be carried out if necessary.

Should the patient develop metastases, treatment of this problem would be the same whether she had or had not been reconstructed.

Mammography can be carried out. A little more effort is needed to obtain a satisfactory mammogram where a prosthesis is present.

7. The Other Breast

The plastic surgeon undertaking reconstructive surgery thoroughly realizes that in many cases it is necessary for him to operate on the remaining breast to produce similiarity in size and shape.

While it is perfectly possible for the ablative surgeon to watch the other breast in his patients, the plastic surgeon is not allowed this luxury.

The treatment of the remaining breast, of course, falls into three categories. It may be left alone if it is small and reconstruction of the mastectomy side can be made to approach it in size. Second, it may be elevated and reduced, or third, a prophylactic mastectomy can be carried out first and then reconstruction bilaterally completed in about 6 months.

I personally speak with each woman who comes in for consultation for reconstruction concerning the possibility first of a prophylactic mastectomy of the remaining breast. I go over with her the statistics as they are known today concerning the development of cancer in one breast and development of cancer in the second breast. This is, of course, a difficult discussion, and all factors should be taken into consideration.

The response is usually one of two. The woman will turn to me in distress and state, "How can I lose my other breast, it's the only one that I have left." If this is her reaction, there is no need to proceed any further with the discussion. However, some patients, especially the younger ones, will appreciate the fact that the subject has been brought up. Some state that they understand the problem and feel like it is waiting for the other shoe to drop in expecting cancer to develop on the other side. It is these women with whom a prophylactic mastectomy is discussed in detail, and a number of them will accept the surgery. This decision is the same as the one that must be made by the high-risk woman who is to be considered for a prophylactic mastectomy, and she will be discussed in Chapter 7.

8. Conclusion

Today, any woman who has a mastectomy can be reconstructed. The methods of surgery at our disposal make it possible to reconstruct the woman who had had a modified mastectomy, radical mastectomy, or even an extended radical mastectomy.

Whether these women should undergo reconstruction is another question altogether. To make an intelligent decision, the woman must have input from her ablative surgeon, a plastic surgeon, and a chemotherapist if she is being treated by one.

However, in the long run, it is the woman who must choose the quality of life she desires. Basically, if understanding her problem she chooses reconstruction, it is not for us to refuse it.

No doubt, methods of reconstruction will be refined in the future. It is our belief as plastic surgeons that we in no way jeopardize the survival of the woman.

We hope that we can influence the ablative surgeon to place his incisions better so that the scars will be covered by a normal bra and to leave as much skin and subcutaneous tissue as he feels is safe so that reconstruction in the future will be easier. In addition, we hope that by making reconstruction possible the fear of breast cancer and its resulting mutilizations will be lessened and that women will come in at an earlier time for treatment of their disease.

9. Reading List

1. W. M. Cocke, Jr., *Breast Reconstruction Following Mastectomy for Carcinoma*, Little, Brown, Boston (1977).
2. J. M. Converse, J. G. McCarthy, and J. W. Littler, *Reconstructive Plastic Surgery*, W. B. Saunders, Philadelphia (1977).
3. H. S. Gallager, *Early Breast Cancer: Detection and Treatment*, John Wiley, New York (1975).
4. N. G. Georgiade, *Breast Reconstruction Following Mastectomy*, C. V. Mosby, St. Louis (1979).
5. N. G. Georgiade, *Reconstructive Breast Surgery*, C. V. Mosby, St. Louis (1976).
6. R. M. Goldwyn, *Plastic and Reconstructive Surgery of the Breast*, Little, Brown, Boston (1976).
7. H. P. Leis, Jr., *Diagnosis and Treatment of Breast Lesions*, Medical Examination Publishing Co., Flushing, New York (1970).
8. R. K. Snyderman, Plastic and reconstructive breast surgery, *Am. Fam. Physician*, p. 146 (October 1979).
9. R. K. Snyderman and R. H. Guthrie, Reconstruction of the female breast following radical mastectomy, *Plast. Reconstr. Surg.* **47**, 565 (1971).
10. R. K. Snyderman, *Symposium on Neoplastic and Reconstructive Problems of the Female Breast*, C. V. Mosby, St. Louis (1973).
11. R. K. Snyderman, On breast reconstruction after mastectomy for cancer (editorial), *Plast. Reconstr. Surg.* **57**(2), 224–226 (1976).
12. R. K. Snyderman, The Present Status of Breast Reconstruction Following Mastectomy in the Female, *Aesthetic Plast. Surg.* **3**, 79–85 (1979).
13. R. K. Snyderman, H. S. Gallagher, H. P. Leis, Jr., and J. A. Urban, *The Breast*, C. V. Mosby, St. Louis (1978).

7

The High-Risk Woman

REUVEN K. SNYDERMAN

At a recent national meeting of the American Cancer Society attended by 3000 women, the question was put to the audience by a speaker as to whether or not they follow the routine of breast self-examination. About half the women present raised their hands. Of this group, a number raised the question that they had multiple lumps in their breasts and really were unable to judge whether there was any change from month to month. The advice given these women was that they should not examine their breasts at all.

With more emphasis being given to the early detection of breast cancer and women becoming more knowledgeable about this problem, what can be truly done for the woman who is in a high-risk category?

A woman is at high risk if she falls into any of the following categories:

1. Family history of breast cancer
2. Frequent detection of masses that need biopsies
3. Pathology report indicating a premalignant lesion, such as significant epithelial abnormality of ducts or lobules rated as "borderline"
4. Carcinoma in the other breast
5. Inexorable concern about known premalignant lesions
6. High-risk mammographic pattern if supported by tissue evaluation showing epithelial hyperplasia

Obviously, a woman may fall in a number of these categories but not in all of them, and some may be of more importance than the others.

It is extremely difficult to counsel the woman who sits before you

REUVEN K. SNYDERMAN • College of Medicine/Dentistry of New Jersey–Rutgers Medical School, University Heights, Piscataway, New Jersey 08854.

and gives a history of breast cancer in her family and who has had a number of biopsies and continues to form additional masses.

It is perfectly legitimate and acceptable to advise her to continue to carry out breast self-examination, to be seen twice a year by a competent physician interested in breast cancer, and to have diagnostic aids such as mammograms whenever he feels this is necessary. This conservative method of management is acceptable, but will not prevent a number of these women from developing breast cancer.

Over the past ten years, a number of operations have been developed in the attempt to help the woman in the high-risk group and perhaps prevent her development of breast cancer. These operations can all be considered prophylactic in nature.

It is well known that no operation will remove 100% of the breast tissue. This even includes the so-called radical mastectomy and extended radical mastectomy. What, then, can be offered? An operation called the subcutaneous mastectomy has been developed. Basically, this was an attempt to remove breast tissue, leaving the skin envelope and the areolar and nipple complex in tact. Some surgeons carry out a most meticulous dissection and probably can remove a great deal of the breast tissue. Others, in order to produce a better-looking breast, will skimp on the dissection, leaving thick skin flaps with much breast tissue behind.

Work done by Goldwyn on cadavers and Snyderman on patients has shown that even after a careful subcutaneous mastectomy, breast tissue can be found by biopsy in the subclavicular area, in the postauricular nipple area, and in the axillary area.

An operation called a prophylactic mastectomy has also been developed (see Fig. 1). While this procedure does not remove 100% of the breast tissue, it appears to be able to give both the operative surgeon and the patient some feeling of security.

The patient is brought to the operating room with her bra on. This is outlined on the chest wall. The areolar nipple area is then marked with a washer, and lines of excision are indicated. Depending on the size of the breast, more or less skin can be removed. The patient is then placed in the akimbo position on the operating table, and the chest is prepped and draped under general anesthesia. The areolar nipple complex is removed and placed in a saline sponge on the surgical table to be used later in the surgical procedure. The skin marked previously is not excised, and a complete dissection of the breast including the gland, the tail of the breast, and the lower axillary nodes is carried out. On completion of the operation, there is a clean field similar in appearance to that following a modified or radical mastectomy. After careful hemostasis is obtained, the flaps may be approximated or even overlapped by removing some epithelium if extra skin is available.

The areolar nipple complex is thinned to that of a split thickness graft, and if the chest wall flaps appear viable, the areolar nipple complex may be returned to its proper position making use of a bolus technique. If there is some question as to the viability on the chest wall, then the areolar nipple complex can be temporarily banked in the inguinal area. Drains are usually inserted before completion of the operation, and a large pressure dressing is applied.

The drains may be removed in 2 days, and while some serous fluid may collect, healing is usually uneventful.

Approximately 6 months later, when the skin is again movable over the chest wall, silicone implants may be inserted, and if an areolar nipple complex is needed, it can be constructed then or at a later date.

The insertion of an implant immediately after a prophylactic mastectomy is not a safe procedure because if the flaps have been cut thin enough, there is the possibility that the implant will extrude through the incision or other scarred areas.

The patient who considers this type of surgery must be given a careful description of what is to be done. If possible, she should see postoperative photographs, and she must understand that her final result will hardly be a cosmetic result. Obviously, there are not a great number of patients who are candidates for this procedure. It is difficult to suggest this operation to a young woman. Usually, the surgery becomes acceptable to them after they have had years of difficulty with masses.

Normally, the best approach is to explain the procedure in detail and allow the woman to make up her mind concerning the procedure. If she has had a number of biopsies, she may well choose to wait until another biopsy is necessary before agreeing to the prophylactic mastectomy.

Each time the patient has had a biopsy, it is well to have the specimen carefully examined, and any signs of premalignant change will aid one in advising a prophylactic mastectomy.

When the breast tissue is removed in a prophylactic mastectomy, it should be carefully examined in the pathology laboratory with the help of specimen radiography. Should cancer of an *in situ* nature be found, then probably no further surgery is indicated. If an invasive carcinoma is found, then one should consider a more thorough axillary dissection.

In summary, prophylactic mastectomy is an operation that should be considered for the high-risk woman. As of today, this operation should be used only in a small number of women. It will take a number of years until statistics show whether this approach to the prevention of breast cancer is an acceptable one.

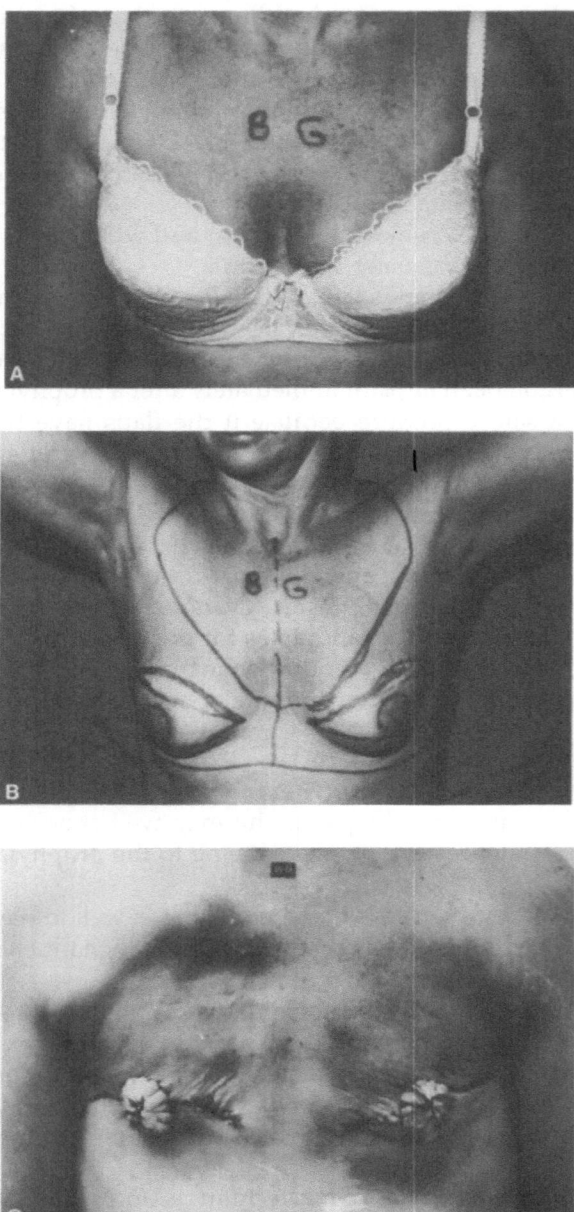

Fig. 1. (A) Patient (who had had nine biopsies) in the operating room with the bra in position. (B) Preoperative markings in the operating room showing the outline of the bra, areolar nipple complex to be removed, and areas of skin excision. (C) Early postoperative

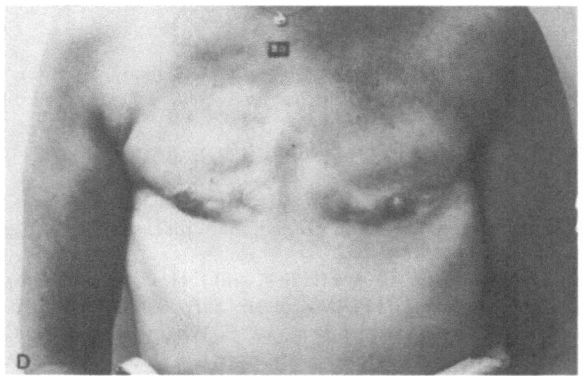

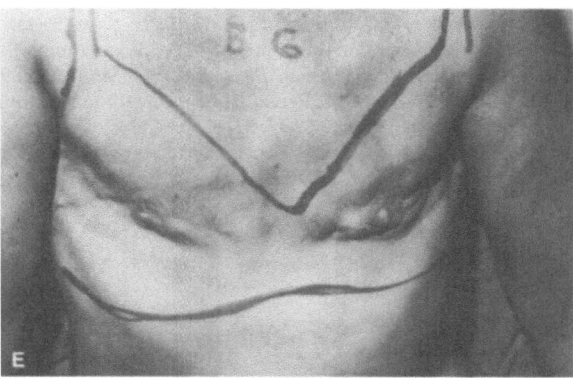

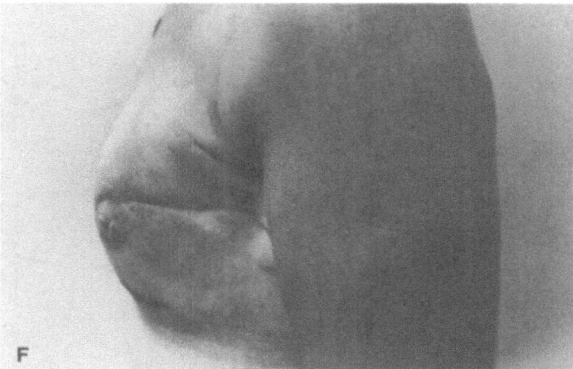

view showing areolar nipple complexes replaced on the chest wall. (D) Late postoperative view. (E) Patient in the operating room. The bra is outlined on the chest wall ready for insertion of the prosthesis. (F) Early postoperative view showing insertion of the prosthesis.

Reading List

1. N. J. Georgiade, *Reconstructive Breast Surgery*, C. V. Mosby, St. Louis (1976).
2. R. M. Goldwyn, *Plastic and Reconstructive Surgery of the Breast*, Little, Brown, Boston (1976).
3. R. M. Goldwyn, Subcutaneous mastectomy: Perspectives and problems, *J. Med. Soc. N. J.* **74**,(2), 1050–1052 (1977).
4. B. S. Freeman and D. R. Wiemer, Total glandular mastectomy: Modifications of the subcutaneous mastectomy for use in premalignant disease of the breast, *Plast. Reconstr. Surg.* **62**(2), 167–172 (1978).
5. C. E. Horton, J. E. Adamson, R. A. Mladick, and J. H. Carraway, Simple mastectomy with immediate reconstruction, *Plast. Reconstr. Surg.* **53**(1), 42–47 (1974).
6. K. S. McCarty, Jr., G. H. D. Kresterson, W. E. Wilkinson, and N. Georgiade, Histopathologic study of subcutaneous mastectomy specimens from patients with carcinoma of the contralateral breast, *Surg. Gynecol. Obstet.* 147(5), 682–688 (1978).
7. E. E. Peacock, Jr., Biological basis for management of benign disease of the breast: The case against subcutaneous mastectomy, *J. Plast. Reconstr. Surg.* **55**(1), 14–20 (1975).
8. V. R. Pennisi and A. Capozzi, The incidence of obscure carcinoma in subcutaneous mastectomy: Results of a national survey, *Plast. Reconstr. Surg.* **56**(1) 9–12 (1975).
9. V. R. Pennisi, A. Capozzi, and F. M. Perez, Subcutaneous mastectomy data: A preliminary report, *Plast. Reconstr. Surg.* **59**(1), 53–56 (1977).
10. A. B. Redfern and J. E. Hoopes, Subcutaneous mastectomy: A plea for conservatism, *Plast. Reconstr. Surg.* **62**(5), 706–707 (1978).

8

Comparative Pathological Study of Breast Carcinoma among American and Japanese Women

GOI SAKAMOTO, HARUO SUGANO, and
WILLIAM H. HARTMANN

1. Introduction

Breast carcinoma among Japanese females is characterized by a relatively low incidence and good prognosis.[6] The recent annual death rate due to breast carcinoma among Japanese females is 5 per 100,000. This death rate is about one sixth of that among American females. According to *Cancer Incidence in Five Continents,*[2] the annual incidence of breast cancer per 100,000 Japanese females ranged from 12.1 in Osaka Prefecture to 16.6 in Okayama Prefecture. This incidence is very low when compared with that of American females. In Connecticut, the incidence is 71.7 per 100,000 females.

In this study, we have investigated in detail both Japanese and American patients with breast carcinoma by comparing the histological distribution and 10-year survival rate of breast-carcinoma patients of the Cancer Institute Hospital (CIH), Tokyo, Japan, and the Vanderbilt University Hospital (VUH), Nashville, Tennessee.

GOI SAKAMOTO • Department of Pathology, Cancer Institute, Tokyo 170, Japan.   HARUO SUGANO • Cancer Institute, Tokyo 170, Japan.   WILLIAM H. HARTMANN • Department of Pathology, Vanderbilt University Hospital, Nashville, Tennessee 37232.

2. Material and Methods

We used 2604 breast-carcinoma cases treated at the CIH between 1956 and 1975 and 755 cases treated at the VUH between 1956 and 1976. For the comparative study of 10-year survival rates, we used only those cases treated by radical mastectomy and followed more than 10 years from operation: 936 cases from the CIH between 1956 and 1965 and 320 cases from the VUH between 1956 and 1967.

All specimens of both hospitals were reviewed by one of the authors (G.S.) and classified using the Japanese classification of breast carcinoma.

2.1. Tumor Size and Lymph-Node Metastasis

In this study, the size of the tumor is the largest diameter of the tumor measured on the cut surface of the gross specimen as recorded in the pathology report.

Lymph-node metastasis, using the "n" classification, was grouped from n0 to n3. Based on histological examination of lymph nodes, we classified them as follows:

n0: no metastasis
$n1\alpha$: 1–3 positive axillary lymph nodes
$n1\beta$: 4 or more positive axillary lymph nodes
n2: metastasis in subclavicular lymph nodes
n3: metastasis in supraclavicular lymph nodes

2.2. Ten-Year Survival Rate

In calculating survival rate, the following method of computation was used:

Ten-year survival rate = number of cases surviving more than 10 years/number of cases followed up for more than 10 years, × 100.

3. Histological Classification

Each case was classified according to the histological classification of breast carcinoma that has been used in the Department of Pathology, Cancer Institute, Tokyo, and adopted by the Japan Mammary Cancer Society.[3] This classification is fundamentally the same as the WHO classification with a subclassification of the common breast-cancer types (see Table I).

Table I
Histological Classification and Case Distribution

Classification	CIH (1956–1975) Number of cases	%	VUH (1956–1976): R+S+Bx[a] Number of cases	%
I. Noninfiltrating carcinoma				
Ductal	72 ⎫		15 ⎫	
Lobular *in situ*	7 ⎬ 9	3.5	21 ⎬ 44	5.8
Paget's[b]	11 ⎭		8 ⎭	
II. Infiltrating carcinoma				
A. Common type				
Papillotubular	545	20.9	80	10.6
Medullary tubular	520	20.0	113	15.0
Scirrhous	1248	47.9	410	54.3
B. Special type				
Mucous	93	3.6	28	3.7
Medullary with lymphoid infiltration	50	1.9	9	1.2
Lobular	54	2.1	68	9.0
Squamous cell	3	0.12	2	0.26
Carcinosarcoma	1	0.04	1	0.13
TOTALS	2604		755	

[a](R): Radical mastectomy (596 cases); (S) simple mastectomy (90 cases); (Bx) biopsy (69 cases).
[b]Paget's carcinoma means Paget's disease with noninfiltrating ductal carcinoma.

According to this classification, breast carcinoma is divided into two major categories: noninfiltrating and infiltrating. Infiltrating carcinoma is further classified into common type and special type. Infiltrating common-type carcinoma has three subgroups: papillotubular carcinoma, medullary tubular carcinoma, and scirrhous carcinoma. Papillotubular carcinoma is characterized by the projection of papillae into glandular lumina and includes papillary and comedo carcinoma. Medullary tubular carcinoma is a solid tumor mass consisting of tubular or trabecular structures with expansive growth compressing the surrounding tissue and forming a sharp border. Scirrhous carcinoma is characterized by cancer nests or cells accompanied by marked fibrosis. The classification of common type is based on the predominant one when there are two or three different histological types. When there are equal amounts of different histological types, the one with the worst prognosis determines the classification.

4. Results

4.1. Case Distribution

4.1.1. Histological Type

The case distribution by histological type is shown in Table I.

The CIH cases had 3.5% noninfiltrating carcinoma, 88.8% infiltrating carcinoma common types, and 7.7% infiltrating carcinoma special type. The VUH cases had 5.8% noninfiltrating carcinoma, 79.9% infiltrating carcinoma common type, and 14.3% infiltrating carcinoma special type.

a. Noninfiltrating Carcinomas. When the noninfiltrating carcinomas are compared as a group, there is no significant difference of incidence between the CIH (3.5%) and the VUH (5.8%). There is a significant difference of incidence when subgroups are compared within the noninfiltrating carcinomas. Within this group, the ratio of noninfiltrating ductal carcinoma at the CIH (80%; 72 of 90 patients) is much higher than that at the VUH (34%; 15 of 44 patients), but the ratio of lobular carcinoma *in situ* at the VUH (44.7%; 21 of 44 patients) is much higher than that at the CIH (7.8%; 7 of 90 patients).

b. Infiltrating Carcinomas. In infiltrating carcinoma common type, the incidence of papillotubular carcinoma shows a remarkable difference between the CIH (20.9%) and the VUH (10.6%). In infiltrating carcinoma special type, the incidence of infiltrating lobular carcinoma at the CIH (2.1%) is lower than that at the VUH (9.0%). It is noteworthy that the incidence of lobular carcinoma, both *in situ* and infiltrating, among Japanese females is distinctly lower than that among American females, and the incidence of noninfiltrating ductal carcinoma and papillotubular carcinoma among Japanese females is much higher than that among American females.

4.1.2. Age at Operation

Breast-cancer incidence among Japanese females has a peak at ages 40–49, whereas among American females it has a peak at ages 50–59 (Table II and Fig. 1). There is a gap of one decade when the peak age is compared between breast-carcinoma patients at the CIH and the VUH. As shown in Fig. 1, the age distribution of patients at the CIH has a sharp and narrow curve with a striking peak at ages 40–49. On the other hand, that at the VUH has a gently sloping and wide curve with a rounded peak at ages 50–59. At the VUH, the patients were distributed

Table II
Case Distribution by Age at Operation

Age at operation	CIH (1956–1975)		VUH (1956–1976): R+S+Bx[a]	
	Number of cases	%	Number of cases	%
20–29	38	1.5	2	0.3
30–39	464	17.8	59	7.8
40–49	1057	40.6	160	21.2
50–59	650	25.0	191	25.3
60–69	281	10.8	162	21.5
70–79	107	4.1	128	17.0
≥80	7	0.3	53	7.0
TOTALS	2604		755	
Premenopausal	1550	59.5	315	41.7
Postmenopausal	1054	40.5	440	58.3
TOTALS	2604		755	

[a]See Table I, footnote a.

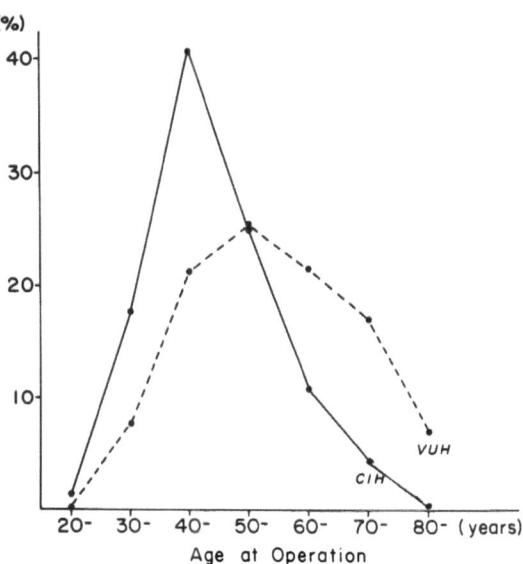

Fig. 1. Case distribution by age at operation.

almost evenly by decades: 40–49 (21.2%), 50–59 (25.3%), and 60–69 (21.5%) years of age.

The ratio of premenopausal to postmenopausal patients is 6:4 (CIH) and 4:6 (VUH), respectively. These age distributions show that breast carcinoma is most frequent among middle-aged females in Japan and elder females in the United States.

4.1.3. Size of Tumor

Case distribution by tumor size shows no significant difference between the CIH and the VUH (Table III). In detail, the ratio of patients who have smaller-sized tumors, such as less than 2 cm in greatest diameter, is 6% higher at the CIH, and the ratio of patients who have larger-sized tumors is 10% higher at the VUH. In other words, on an average, the tumor size of breast carcinoma among Japanese females is slightly smaller than that among American females.

4.1.4. Lymph-Node Metastasis

The ratio of case distribution of lymph nodes without metastasis is almost the same in patients of the CIH (53.7%) and the VUH (54.9%) (Table IV). This also means that the ratio of lymph nodes with metastasis is almost the same.

As shown in Table IV, at the CIH, many patients underwent subclavicular or supraclavicular lymph-node dissection or both, but at the VUH, lymph-node dissections are limited to an axillary group in almost all patients.

The rates of $n1\alpha$ are almost equal at the CIH (24.0%) and the VUH (24.5%). The incidence of $n1\beta$ at the VUH (20.6%) is much higher than that at the CIH (8.0%), but after the sum of the number of $n1\beta$, n2, and

Table III
Case Distribution by Size of Tumor

Size of tumor	CIH (1956–1975)		VUH (1956–1976): R+S[a]	
	Number of cases	%	Number of cases	%
<2 cm	1167	44.8	244	38.8
2.1–5 cm	1226	47.1	271	43.1
≥5.1 cm	211	8.1	114	18.1
TOTALS	2604		629	

[a]See Table I, footnote *a*.

Table IV
Case Distribution by Lymph-Node Metastasis

Lymph-node metastasis		CIH (1956–1975)		VUH (1956–1976): R[a]	
		Number of cases	%	Number of cases	%
Negative	(n0)	1399	53.7	327	54.9
Axillary 1–3	(n1α)	625	24.0	146	24.5
Axillary 4 or more	(n1β)	209	8.0	123	20.6
Subclavicular	(n2)	298	11.4	—	—
Supraclavicular	(n3)	73	2.8	—	—
TOTALS		2604		596	
Negative		1399	53.7	327	54.9
Positive		1205	46.3	269	45.1
TOTALS		2604		596	

[a]See Table I, footnote a.

n3 patients at the CIH is determined, the ratio (22.2%) is almost the same as that of the n1β at the VUH (20.6%).

4.2. Ten-Year Survival Rate

4.2.1. Histological Type

The 10-year rate of each histological type is shown in Table V.

The over all 10-year survival rate of breast-carcinoma patients treated after radical mastectomy is 63.8% (597 of 936 patients) at the CIH and 46.9% (150 of 320 patients) at the VUH. This indicates that breast cancer among Japanese females has a better prognosis than that among American females.

In patients of every subgroup of infiltrating carcinoma common type, the 10-year survival rate at the CIH is higher than that at the VUH.

Among patients with infiltrating carcinoma common type, papillotubular carcinoma shows the most favorable 10-year survival rate and that of scirrhous carcinoma the worst 10-year survival rate at both institutions. Medullary tubular carcinoma shows an intermediate 10-year survival rate.

Almost all the 10-year survival rates of patients with infiltrating carcinoma special type (except that of lobular carcinoma at the VUH) are higher than those of patients with infiltrating carcinoma common type. There is a significant difference in the 10-year survival rate of patients with infiltrating lobular carcinoma between the CIH (78.6%) and the VUH (45.8%).

Table V
Ten-Year Survival Rates by Histological Classification

Classification	CIH (1956–1965)			VUH (1956–1967): R[a]		
	Number of cases[b]	10-Year survivors[c]	10-Year survival rate (%)	Number of cases[b]	10-Year survivors	10-Year survival rate (%)
I. Noninfiltrating carcinoma						
Ductal	36	33	91.7	3	3	100.0
Lobular *in situ*	—	—	—	—	—	—
II. Infiltrating carcinoma						
A. Common type						
Papillotubular	230	168	73.0	32	19	59.4
Medullary tubular	138	79	57.2	51	26	51.0
Scirrhous	457	259	56.7	196	81	41.3
B. Special type						
Mucous	36	27	75.0	6	4	66.7
Medullary with lymphoid infiltration	16	13	81.3	3	3	100.0
Lobular	14	11	78.6	24	11	45.8
Squamous cell	1	0	0.0	1	1	100.0
Carcinosarcoma	0	0	—	1	0	0.0
Paget's	8	7	87.5	3	2	66.7
TOTALS	936	597	63.8	320	150	46.9

[a] See Table 1, footnote a.
[b] Number of cases followed up for more than 10 years.
[c] Number of cases surviving more than 10 years.

4.2.2. Age at Operation

In each age group, the 10-year survival rate at the CIH is higher than that at the VUH (Table VI and Fig. 2).

The patients of both the CIH and the VUH in the age groups 30–39, 40–49, and 50–59 years of age show a favorable prognosis.

At the CIH, the 10-year survival rate of premenopausal patients is 66.4% (366 of 551 patients) and that of postmenopausal patients is 60.0% (231 of 385 patients). The difference in the 10-year survival rate between premenopausal and postmenopausal patients is only 6.4%. On the other hand, this difference is 27.2% at the VUH: 61.3% (92 of 150 patients) in premenopausal as compared to 34.1% (58 of 170 patients) in post-menopausal patients. From another viewpoint, there is no significant difference in the 10-year survival rate of the premenopausal group between Japanese and American patients (66.4 vs. 61.3%), but there is a distinct difference (60.0 vs. 34.1%) in the postmenopausal group. In other words, knowing whether an American female breast-carcinoma patient is premenopausal or postmenopausal is critical for prognosis, but it is not critical among Japanese females.

The 10-year survival rate by age at operation of each histological type of the infiltrating carcinoma common type is shown in Fig. 3. By histological type, the patients at both institutions in the age groups 30–39, 40–49, and 50–59 years of age show a favorable prognosis. At the VUH, the patients over 60 with papillotubular carcinoma and scirrhous carcinoma show a relatively poor prognosis. At both the CIH and the VUH, the 10-year survival rate of patients with medullary tubular carcinoma shows no significant difference that is age-related.

4.2.3. Size of Tumor

In each tumor-size group, the 10-year survival rate for patients at the CIH is higher than at the VUH (Table VII and Fig. 4). There are differences in the 10-year survival rate between the patients at the CIH and the VUH with tumors less than 2 cm (80.9% at the CIH vs. 61.2% at the VUH) and with tumors more than 5.1 cm in greatest diameter (39.4% at the CIH vs. 22.4% at the VUH). This difference is rather slight in the patients with tumors 2.1–5 cm in greatest diameter (51.2% at the CIH vs. 47.8% at the VUH).

The 10-year survival rate by tumor size of each histological type of the infiltrating carcinoma common type is shown in Fig. 5. At both institutions, there is a good correlation between prognosis and tumor size in patients with medullary tubular carcinoma and scirrhous carcinoma. The 10-year survival rate of patients with papillotubular car-

Table VI
Ten-Year Survival Rates by Age at Operation

Age at operation	CIH (1956–1965)			VUH (1956–1967): R[a]		
	Number of cases[b]	10-Year survivors[c]	10-Year survival rate (%)	Number of cases[b]	10-Year survivors[c]	10-Year survival rate (%)
20–29	14	7	50.0	0	—	—
30–39	194	125	64.7	38	21	55.3
40–49	347	234	67.4	74	47	63.5
50–59	261	168	64.4	75	41	54.7
60–69	86	48	55.8	79	28	35.4
70–79	34	15	44.1	41	13	31.7
≥80	0			13	0	0.0
TOTALS	936	597	63.8	320	150	46.9
Premenopausal	551	366	66.4	150	92	61.3
Postmenopausal	385	231	60.0	170	58	34.1
TOTALS	936			320		

[a] See Table I, footnote *a*.
[b,c] See Table V, footnotes *b* and *c*.

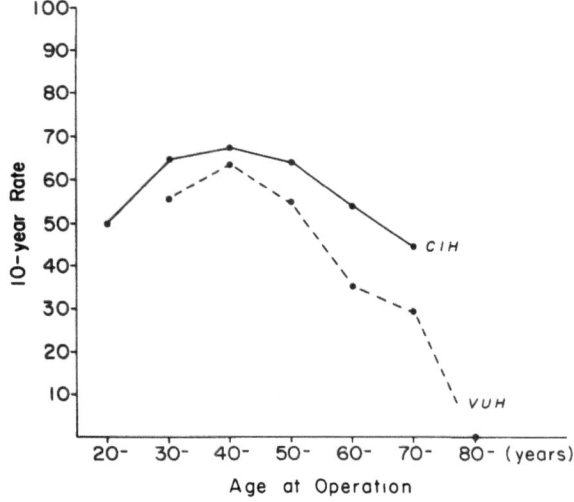

Fig. 2. Ten-year survival rates by age at operation.

cinoma shows no significant difference by tumor size. The 10-year survival rates of patients with medullary tubular carcinoma and scirrhous carcinoma in the group with tumors 2.1–5 cm are slightly higher at the VUH than those at the CIH.

4.2.4. Lymph-Node Status

In each group of patients with lymph nodes containing metastases, the 10-year survival rate at the CIH (42.2%) is higher than at the VUH

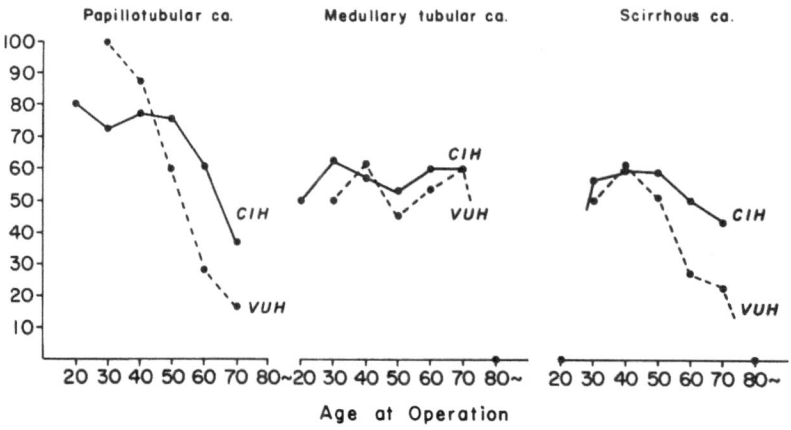

Fig. 3. Ten-year survival rates of each histological type by age at operation.

Table VII

Ten-Year Survival Rates by Size of Tumor

Size of tumor	CIH (1956–1965)			VUH (1956–1967): R^a		
	Number of cases[b]	10-Year survivors[c]	10-Year survival rate (%)	Number of cases[b]	10-Year survivors[c]	10-Year survival rate (%)
<2 cm	424	343	80.9	107	65	61.2
2.1–5 cm	441	226	51.2	134	64	47.8
≥5.1 cm	71	28	39.4	49	11	22.4
Unclear	—	—	—	30	10	—
TOTALS	936	597	63.8	320	150	46.9

[a] See Table I, footnote *a*.
[b,c] See Table V, footnotes *b* and *c*.

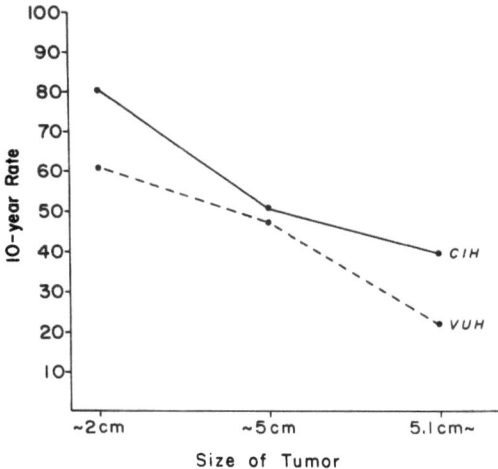

Fig. 4. Ten-year survival rates by size of tumor.

(28.8%) (Table VIII and Fig. 6). The 10-year survival rates in the patients with no lymph-node metastasis are 82.6% (CIH) and 64.0% (VUH).

In the Japanese patients, there is a considerable difference in the 10-year survival rate between $n1\alpha$ and $n1\beta$. In other words, it is critical for prognosis to know whether a Japanese patient has fewer or more than four positive lymph nodes. In the American patients, it seems that the critical point is whether or not a patient has lymph-node metastases.

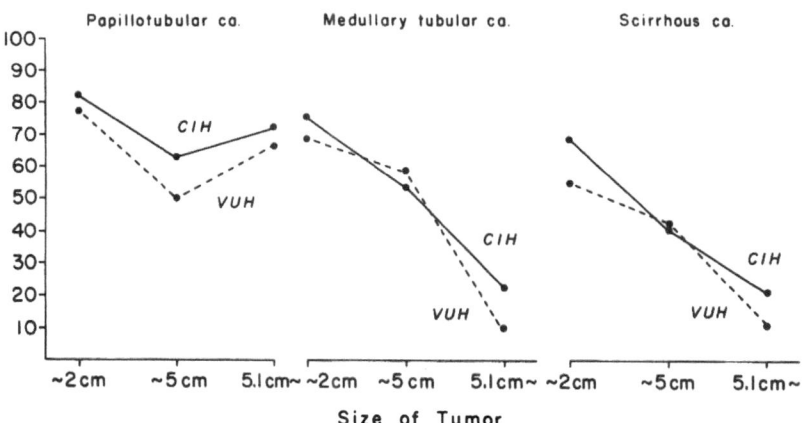

Fig. 5. Ten-year survival rates of each histological type by tumor size.

Table VIII
Ten-Year Survival Rates by Lymph-Node Metastasis

Lymph-node metastasis		CIH (1956–1965)			VUH (1956–1967): R[a]		
		Number of cases[b]	10-Year survivors[c]	10-Year survival rate (%)	Number of cases[b]	10-Year survivors[c]	10-Year survival rate (%)
Negative	(n0)	500	413	82.6	164	105	64.0
Axillary 1–3	(n1α)	234	138	59.0	95	32	33.7
Axillary 4 or more	(n1β)	63	19	30.2	61	13	21.3
Subclavicular	(n2)	116	24	20.7	—	—	—
Subclavicular	(n3)	23	3	13.0	—	—	—
TOTALS		936	597	63.8	320	150	46.9
Negative		500	413	82.6	164	105	64.0
Positive		436	184	42.2	156	45	28.8
TOTALS		936			320		

[a] See Table I, footnote a.
[b,c] See Table V, footnotes b and c.

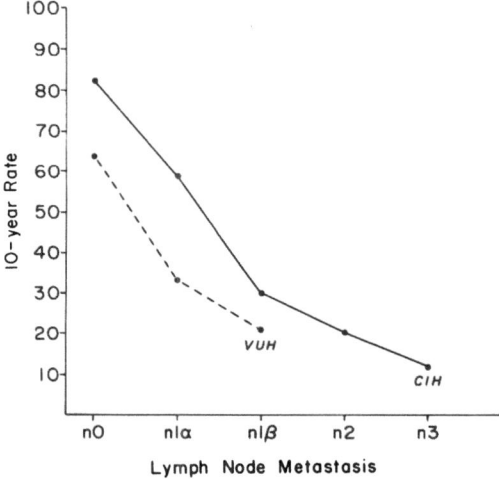

Fig. 6. Ten-year survival rates by lymph-node metastasis.

The 10-year survival rates by lymph-node metastasis of the infiltrating carcinoma common type are shown in Fig. 7. In each histological type, lymph-node metastasis is clearly correlated with the prognosis. In patients with scirrhous carcinoma, the 10-year survival rate of the n0 group at the VUH (58.9%) is almost equal to the 10-year survival rate of the n1α group at the CIH (57.5%), the n1α at the VUH (33.3%) to the n1β at the CIH (31.6%), and the n1β at the VUH (16.3%) to the n2 at the CIH (14.8%).

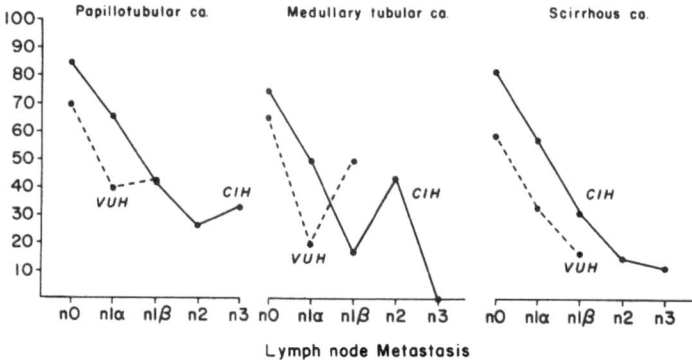

Fig. 7. Ten-year survival rates of each histological type by lymph-node metastasis.

5. Discussion

It is noteworthy that the incidence of lobular carcinoma, both *in situ* and infiltrating, among Japanese females is distinctly lower than that among American females. Furthermore, as already mentioned, there is a significant difference in the 10-year survival rates of patients with infiltrating lobular carcinoma at the CIH (78.6%) and the VUH (45.8%). After equalizing for the size of tumor and presence of lymph-node metastasis, the 10-year survival rates of patients with infiltrating lobular carcinoma at the VUH are lower than those at the CIH (Table IX).

The incidence of lobular carcinoma in Japan is very low and is significantly different from the incidence in the Western countries. However, Sugano and Sakamoto[7] found that the incidence of lobular carcinoma among Japanese females has gradually increased. At the CIH, before 1965, the incidence of infiltrating lobular carcinoma was around 1% of all breast cancers, from 1971 to 1975 it was 3.4%, and most recently, for 1974–1975, it has increased to 5.3%. Therefore, it may be said that the incidence of infiltrating lobular carcinoma among Japanese females is gradually approaching that of American females.

There is a significant difference with reference to the age distribution of breast carcinoma between Japanese and American females. Breast-carcinoma incidence among Japanese females has a peak at ages 40–49 and decreases sharply past age 60, whereas among American females, the rate continues to increase through the 7th and 8th decades. The explanation for this difference remains obscure, but is deserving of further study.

Japanese female breast-carcinoma patients have a better prognosis as compared with American females. This is true when they are examined in detail after equalizing for tumor size (see Fig. 4) or presence of lymph-node metastasis (see Fig. 6). As already mentioned, at the VUH, lymph-node dissections are limited to the axillia in almost all patients. If we combine the CIH patients of the n0, n1α, and n1β groups, the overall 10-year survival rate becomes 71.0% (570 of 797 patients). Then the difference of the overall 10-year survival rate becomes 24.1% between the CIH (71.0%) and the VUH (46.9%). There must be several factors causing this remarkable difference in survival, but almost all causes originate from the distinctive difference of prognosis between premenopausal and postmenopausal patients among American females. Furthermore, among American females the incidence of carcinoma among postmenopausal women is much higher than that among premenopausal women. In patients with breast carcinoma among American females, the difference in the 10-year survival rate between premenopausal and postmenopausal patients is 27.2%. On the other hand, this difference

Table IX
Ten-Year Survival Rates of Infiltrating Lobular Carcinoma

Parameter	CIH (1956–1965)			VUH (1956–1967): R[a]		
	Number of cases[b]	10-Year survivors[c]	10-Year survival rate (%)	Number of cases[b]	10-Year survivors	10-Year survival rate (%)
Size of tumor						
< 2 cm	7	6	85.7	5	3	60.0
2.1–5 cm	6	5	83.3	10	5	50.0
≥ 5.1 cm	1	0	0.0	6	3	50.0
TOTALS	14	11	78.6	24	11	45.8
Lymph-node metastasis						
Negative (n0)	7	6	85.7	12	8	66.7
Axillary 1–3 (n1α)	5	4	80.0	7	2	28.6
Axillary 4 or more (n1β)	—	—	—	5	1	20.0
Subclavicular (n2)	2	1	50.0	—	—	—
TOTALS	14	11	78.6	24	11	45.8

[a]See Table I, footnote a.
[b,c]See Table V, footnotes b and c.

Table X

Premenopausal and Postmenopausal Ten-Year Survival Rates by Tumor Size and Lymph-Node Metastasis: VUH (1956–1967)

Parameter	Premenopausal			Postmenopausal		
	Number of cases[a] (%)	10-Year survivors[b]	10-Year survival rate (%)	Number of cases[a] (%)	10-Year survivors[b]	10-Year survival rate (%)
Size of tumor						
< 2 cm	55 (40.4)	41	74.5	52 (33.8)	24	46.2
2.1–5 cm	59 (43.4)	39	66.1	75 (48.7)	25	33.3
≥ 5.1 cm	22 (16.2)	6	27.3	27 (17.5)	4	14.8
Unclear	14 —	6	—	16 —	4	—
TOTALS	150	92	61.3	170	58	34.1
Lymph-node metastasis						
Negative (n0)	80 (53.8)	63	78.8	84 (49.4)	42	50.0
Axillary 1–3 (n1α)	45 (30.0)	21	46.7	50 (29.4)	11	22.0
Axillary 4 or more (n1β)	25 (16.7)	8	32.0	36 (21.2)	5	13.9
TOTALS	150	92	61.3	170	58	34.1

[a,b]See Table V, footnotes *b* and *c*.

among Japanese females is only 6.4%. Of significance is our observation that the 10-year survival rates of all premenopausal breast-carcinoma patients at both institutions are almost equal (Fig. 8).

As shown in Table X, when case distributions between pre-menopausal and postmenopausal groups at the VUH are compared, the incidence of patients with negative lymph nodes and smaller-sized tumors (such as less than 2 cm in greatest diameter) is slightly greater in the premenopausal group. Those with axillary lymph-node metastasis and with large-sized tumors (such as more than 5.1 cm in greatest diameter) are more common in the postmenopausal group. This suggests that American postmenopausal breast-carcinoma patients have slightly larger tumors and more lymph-node metastasis than pre-menopausal patients. This is not sufficient to explain the difference in the 10-year survival rate between premenopausal and postmenopausal patients, the rate being distinctly lower in the postmenopausal patients. The explanation for this difference remains a problem, but the data presented above show that among American females, postmenopausal breast carcinoma is more malignant than premenopausal breast carcinoma.

There have been other studies comparing pathological features of breast cancer between a Japanese and an American population. [4,5,8] These studies are not completely comparable to this one for some very significant reasons. All previous studies utilized classifications of breast carcinoma that are in common use in the United States. This study utilizes a classification system for breast carcinoma that is used in Japan. The primary difference is the attempt by the Japanese to subdivide the infiltrating duct cell carcinoma, which makes up the largest group of breast carcinoma in the United States. The previous studies were also

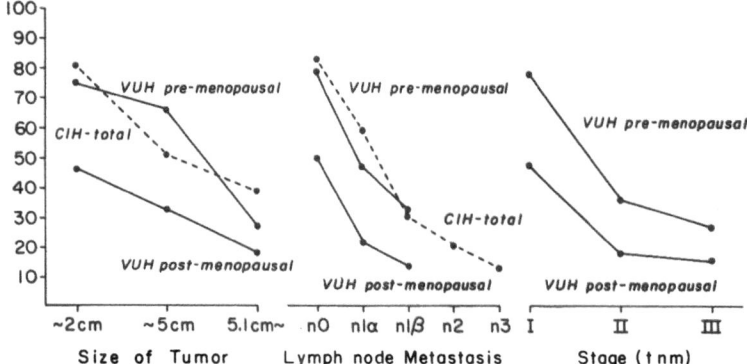

Fig. 8. Premenopausal and postmenopausal ten-year survival rates by tumor size, lymph-node metastasis, and stage.

Table XI
Percentage of All Cancers

	Colloid Carcinoma		Intraductal Carcinoma	
Ref. No.	American	Japanese	American	Japanese
4	2.6	4.2	3.8	6.2
5	1.4	3.2	3.8	8.7
8	2.0	5.0	—	—
This study	3.7	3.6	2.0	2.8

concerned primarily with validity of diagnosis as determined by observer reproducibility[4] and fine points of histological observation with survival data[8] and without survival data.[5] The survival data that are given are for 5 years,[8] while this chapter reports 10-year survival data. Histological observations were made by more than one observer, [4,5,8] whereas ours were all made by one observer.

There are, however, useful comparisons that can be made. Comments have been made that colloid (mucous) carcinoma is more common in the Japanese than in the American female. Although criteria for the classification of a case as colloid carcinoma are precisely stated by some, [3,5] it is doubtful that they were so used by all. Nonetheless, our observations leave one to conclude that the higher incidence of colloid (mucous) carcinoma of the breast for the Japanese may no longer be true and perhaps should be investigated further (Table XI).

Similarly, the difference in the incidence of intraductal carcinoma in the two populations also seems to be disappearing (Table XI).

In situ lobular carcinoma is more common in the American than the Japanese female, but even this appears to be changing.[7]

Because of differences in terminology, the medullary carcinomas cannot be compared. There is evidence that this group of carcinomas may be very heterogenous since the term medullary carcinoma is variously used around the world.[1]

6. Conclusion

Breast carcinoma is a very common and a very serious disease. Our observations support others that studies comparing patient populations from different parts of the world can be effectively accomplished and are useful, that previous differences in incidence of certain types of breast carcinoma among these populations may be disappearing, and that as these differences in pathological types of breast carcinoma disappear, carcinoma of the female breast may become, worldwide, a more homogeneous process.

7. References

1. P. Correa and W. D. Johnson (ed.), An international survey of distribution of histologic types of breast cancer, *Union Internationale Centre le Cancer* Technical Report Series, Vol. 35, Geneva (1978).
2. IARC, *Cancer Incidence in Five Continents*, Vol. III, IARC Publications (1976).
3. Japan Mammary Cancer Society, General rule for clinical and histological record of mammary cancer, *Jpn. J. Surg.* **5**, 118–131 (1975).
4. B. MacMahon, A. S. Morrison, L. V. Ackerman, R. Lattes, H. B. Taylor, and S. Yuasa, Histologic characteristic of breast cancer in Boston and Tokyo, *Int. J. Cancer* **11**, 338–344 (1973).
5. P. P. Rosen, R. Ashikari, H. Thaler, S. Ishikawa, T. Hirota, O. Abe, H. Yamamoto, E. J. Beattie, Jr., J. A. Urban, and V. Mike, A comparative study of some pathologic features of mammary carcinoma in Tokyo, Japan, and New York, U.S.A., *Cancer* **39**, 429–434 (1977).
6. G. Sakamoto, H. Sugano, and W. H. Hartmann, Comparative clinicopathological study of breast cancer among Japanese and American women, *Jpn. J. Cancer Clin.* **25**, 161–170 (1979) (in Japanese).
7. H. Sugano and G. Sakamoto, Time trend data of breast cancer in Japan: Clinicopathological findings, *Prev. Med.* **7**, 168–172 (1978).
8. E. L. Wynder, T. Kajitani, J. Kuno, J. C. Lucas, Jr., A. DePalo, and J. Farrow, A comparison of survival rates between American and Japanese patients with breast cancer, *Surg. Gynecol. Obstet.* **117**, 196–200 (1963).

Index